D1622601

DYING WITH EASE

DYING WITH EASE

A Compassionate Guide for Making Wiser End-of-Life Decisions

Jeff Spiess

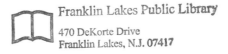
ROWMAN & LITTLEFIELD
Lanham • Boulder • New York • London

This book represents reference material only. It is not intended as a medical manual, and the data presented here are meant to assist the reader in making informed choices regarding wellness. This book is not a replacement for treatment(s) that the reader's personal physician may have suggested. If the reader believes he or she is experiencing a medical issue, professional medical help is recommended. Mention of particular products, companies, or authorities in this book does not entail endorsement by the publisher or author.

Published by Rowman & Littlefield
An imprint of The Rowman & Littlefield Publishing Group, Inc.
4501 Forbes Boulevard, Suite 200, Lanham, Maryland 20706
https://rowman.com

6 Tinworth Street, London SE11 5AL, United Kingdom

British Library Cataloguing in Publication Information Available

Library of Congress Cataloging-in-Publication Data
Names: Spiess, Jeff, 1954– author.
Title: Dying with ease : a compassionate guide for making wiser end-of-life decisions / Jeff Spiess.
Description: Lanham : Rowman & Littlefield, [2020] | Includes bibliographical references and index.
Identifiers: LCCN 2020008601 (print) | LCCN 2020008602 (ebook) | ISBN 9781538141892 (hardcover ; alk. paper) | ISBN 9781538141908 (epub)
Subjects: LCSH: Death—Planning.
Classification: LCC HQ1073 .S6955 2020 (print) | LCC HQ1073 (ebook) | DDC 306.9—dc23
LC record available at https://lccn.loc.gov/2020008601
LC ebook record available at https://lccn.loc.gov/2020008602

♾ ™ The paper used in this publication meets the minimum requirements of American National Standard for Information Sciences Permanence of Paper for Printed Library Materials, ANSI/NISO Z39.48-1992.

For my grandchildren

CONTENTS

INTRODUCTION

If convicted he would be executed, and he fully expected to be found guilty. His trial was a public event, his alleged victims the scions of many of the prominent families of society, including those serving as his prosecutors, judges, and jury. In the seventy years of his life, he had killed no one, betrayed no one, robbed no one, lied to no one, yet he faced capital punishment. The charge was failure to adhere to the religious norms of the land and, in this and other actions, corrupting the youth of the metropolis. The trial jury would be large, perhaps more than five hundred citizens, but it would require only a simple majority for a decision of guilt or innocence. Socrates knew he would die.

The Oracle at Delphi had proclaimed him the wisest of men, though Socrates recognized that any wisdom he possessed lay in the fact that he knew that he did not know. When he thought about death, he said, "To be afraid of death is only another form of thinking that one is wise when one is not. . . . No one knows with regard to death whether it is not really the greatest blessing that can happen to a man; but people dread it as though they were certain that it is the greatest evil."[1]

Socrates died; the jurors who convicted him died; billions of people from his time to ours have died. I will die. You will die. Nobody gets out of here alive. Most of us have some idea of what we think dying will be like and what might happen to us after death. These images come to us from religious teachings, from popular culture, from medical and metaphysical literature, and from our own hopes and fears. But none of this reaches the level of demonstrable fact, at least to those of us who remain alive. If we are honest, we must agree with Socrates that when it comes to what dying is like, what it is all about, we just don't know.

I am a doctor whose patients all die. For most of my life in medical practice, I have been a hospice physician, one whose focus is the care of the dying. Working with the terminally ill is rewarding, fulfilling, frustrating, and humbling, and I, like every self-aware doctor, came to realize that I learn as much from my patients as I did in medical school, and usually these new lessons are more valuable and practical. To me, the most prized of these lessons is the realization that, just like my patients, I will die.

This is a lesson that most people, especially most Americans, have yet to honestly recognize. I am convinced that one of the reasons that conversations and decisions around the end of life are often difficult and frightening is because they occur in foreign and unfamiliar territory. The participants—patients, family members, caregivers, and medical professionals—have not considered death as a personal reality, have not intentionally faced their own mortality. Publicized societal events, like the case of Terri Schiavo in 2005 or the story of Brittany Maynard in 2014, bring issues of death and dying to the public consciousness and generate periods of personal and communal thought and conversation. But most of that deliberation and discussion occurs at the less threatening intellectual or public-policy levels and is easily forgotten.

In his best-selling book, *Being Mortal*, surgeon Atul Gawande chronicles his realization that a patient's death does not represent personal or even professional failure. He put it this way: "Death may be the enemy, but it is also the natural order of things. I knew these truths abstractly, but didn't know them concretely—that they could be truths not just for everyone but also for this person right in front of me, for this person I was responsible for."[2] I can't claim any insight into Dr. Gawande's personal reflections, but in this writing, he did not carry this insight to its natural conclusion, that death is the natural order of things not only for the person in front of him but also for him, the one in the white coat.

In ancient Rome, a conquering hero rode in triumphal procession through the city accompanied in his chariot by a valued slave holding the golden laurel over his head and repeatedly advising him that, even in his greatness, he was only mortal. Of course, each of us, at least intellectually, realizes we will die and knows that we share biology and fate with all humanity. The natural circle of life and death is the force that drives the evolutionary process, making us who we are. Every year, on Ash Wednesday, the faithful in many churches are individually reminded that "you are dust, and to dust you shall return." The Koran tells the faithful that "we have incorporated death in your constitution."[3] Even so, we keep the idea of our personal demise at a distance, as an abstraction. We accept the "terms and conditions" without even thinking about reading the fine print.

What I hope to do for the reader of this volume is to personalize these abstractions, to map this foreign territory, to render it both more familiar and less frightening. We will take two approaches to this cartography: information and contemplation. Information from medical, legal, societal, and religious traditions establishes the topography, charts the possible pathways, and identifies alternate routes for one traveling this country. Contemplation identifies and unpacks the baggage we carry with us as well as the fuel and other resources available to us: our histories, our values, our identities, and our loves, hopes, and fears.

The landscape is set by the basic facts, the nuts and bolts of how dying happens in the United States, what the rules and conventions are. There is a disconnect between what American people say they want at the end of their lives and what actually happens to them. One major cause of this divergence is the difference between thinking about dying as a hypothetical event and honestly facing one's own mortality. In this book, we will focus on dying as a personal process, one that each one of us will experience. The experiences and desires expressed by the dying will illustrate and personalize what becomes important at the end of life. Openly considering our own death requires us to break through the natural defenses of denial and allows us to rationally consider our own wishes for this final phase in our lives.

In the United States, issues surrounding the care of the dying, what is often termed "end-of-life care," are obscured by a vocabulary of unfamiliar terms, such as "advance directives," "palliative care," "hospice," "estate planning," "sanctity of life," "euthanasia," and a host of others. State-to-state variation in legislation and policies about issues such as medical marijuana and medical aid in dying highlight that the options available to an individual vary depending on their zip code. Management of pain and suffering brings its own set of questions that can challenge long-held values and personal priorities. The disaster of the current opioid abuse and overdose epidemic further complicates choices for patients, physicians, regulators, and society. Fortunately, the astounding growth in research about, expertise in, and availability of excellent symptom management and care of the seriously and terminally ill provides a plethora of resources for not only dying well but also continuing to live until we die.

American society values autonomy, that rugged individualism, struggling with adversity and prevailing with one's integrity intact. Much of the legislation and activism around end-of-life issues in this country aims to enhance an individual's ability to make their own choices and, to every degree possible, have those choices realized. The question "It's my life, isn't it?" is that quintessentially American expression of personal freedom. And, of course, our death, like our life, is our own. But we do not live, nor do we die, in a vacuum. There are others, because of personal relationship, like spouses or relatives, or because of regulation, like governments, who make claims on us, and those claims need to be recognized and weighed.

Before I began working with the dying, I assumed religious people would more likely acknowledge their terminal state and would therefore choose quality of life over struggling to live longer, to model acceptance rather than resistance. The reality, though, is exactly the opposite: people who rely on religion to cope with adversity are much more likely to undergo aggressive, even futile, procedures and medical care and are less likely to choose hospice care. How can it be that something we think of as comforting actually leads to increased suffering?

To make good choices for our lives at their ends, we should contemplate what our own dying might be like. Historical, philosophical, and religious traditions provide us with some perspectives, but imagining ourselves as the dying one can bring to light our underlying priorities as well as expose hidden emotions and feelings, hopes, and fears. In speaking with individuals and groups about these issues, I have found that these feelings, often long suppressed, can be quite raw. I believe that opening these emotions to consciousness, as we face our own mortality, is an effective way to identify what is most important. In doing this, we make more thoughtful choices about our own lives. I also believe that in becoming more comfortable with our own impermanence, we can be better listeners and counselors for friends or family facing their own existential questions.

My thoughts and perspectives on death and dying have been largely formed from what I have learned from individuals going through it, particularly my patients. I am greatly indebted to them all and am humbled by the opportunity to include some of their stories in this volume. Some of these I wrote down at the time, and others were enhanced by interviewing survivors; I apologize if certain details are not factually accurate, but I present them to the best of my recall, with thankfulness for what they taught me. Names and other personal details have, of course, been altered for privacy.

Much of what I have written represents my own thoughts and opinions, though largely informed by many wiser than me. For the purposes of this exploration, death is defined as a human biologic term. I will not include prenatal demise as a topic, recognizing that some readers might object to that exclusion. My metaphysical mindset is rooted in Western philosophy and the Christian tradition, though I have found much truth and insight in many other sources and have integrated many of these in the text. The quotations from and allusions to sacred writings arise predominantly from Hebrew and Christian scriptures; this is a result of familiarity, not of preference or chauvinism. What I have written here are my thoughts, and I make no apology for them, though I recognize the vastness of what I have yet to learn. I submit this book as just one contribution to the larger ongoing conversation on human meaning.

In this work, I present the reader with information, context, and a little provocation, in the hope of generating more thoughtful and personal imaginings and conversations about death and dying, especially the end of our own lives. If this occurs, it cannot help but inform larger societal deliberation and perhaps even wiser public policy, but my primary hope is for you, dear reader, to become more informed and at peace regarding your own dying.

I

DYING IN AMERICA

Why should I worry about dying? It's not going to happen in my lifetime!

—Raymond Smullyan

She brought a whole box of tissues, yellow Puffs, as I remember. Most of the girls in the class came similarly prepared. This was a school assignment, an outing for our eleventh-grade American History course. Susan, my girlfriend, had warned me that even though, in her opinion, *Gone with the Wind* was the best movie ever made, she would cry all through it. This was in the early 1970s, decades after the movie's initial release, but it was still making periodic appearances in theaters and had (and still has) a devoted following.

The story of the young Georgia belle Scarlett O'Hara, her wiles and weddings, her schemes and dreams, but mostly her impossible romantic love for Ashley Wilkes, all played out through the carnage, destitution, and death during the Civil War and Reconstruction took a toll on Susan's tissue, and I may have even borrowed one or two. Nearing the final climax, Scarlett, then married to the wealthy blockade runner Rhett Butler, but still in love with Ashley, visits the Wilkeses' home where his beloved wife, Melanie, lay on her death bed. The tissue box, now more than half empty, risked depletion as Melanie told Scarlett to look after Ashley after she was gone and then instructed, regarding Scarlett's own husband, "Captain Butler, be kind to him. He loves you so." Scarlett's world crashed around her as she came to see that Ashley was devoted to his wife and that he had never reciprocated Scarlett's affection. Realizing that Rhett was her true love, she frantically ran home through the misty twilight. But Rhett said that he was leaving, that he didn't give a damn. Susan's tears flowed along with Scarlett's as she wept for her losses and then as she brightened to utter that perhaps most maudlin final movie line, "Tomorrow is another day!" The theater lights came on, the tissue box was empty, and a high school class stepped out into the late-afternoon sunshine.

Americans are divided in how they think they would like to die. Some say that they would prefer a sudden and unanticipated ending, with no prolonged time of suffering, just alive one minute and dead the next. For most, though, the idyllic though unrealistic scene of Melanie Hamilton, lying in a darkened room, immaculately clean in a feather bed with down pillows and rich linens, being constantly attended to, comes close to the picture of what they would like their own dying moments to look like. The appeal of this image of one's own dying is the ability to give final advice, express love that will survive, and say good-bye to beloved friends and family. I suspect that these spur-of-the-moment ideas change as an individual's life circumstances alter, as children are born, relationships flourish and dissolve, gains and losses are experienced. Our thoughts about our own death, when we think about it at all, usually come up with a scenario that minimizes suffering, our own and that of those we care about. We want a "good death."

WHAT IS A GOOD DEATH?

A good death is one in which pain and suffering are minimized and which matches the preferences of the dying person and their family. An astute social worker once told me that people die the way they lived. People describe their idealized image of dying with phrases like "death with dignity," "quality of life over quantity of life," and "letting nature take its course." Multiple studies and surveys have fleshed out the details of what this good death actually looks like.

First of all, most Americans say they want to die at home. Home might be peaceful, or it might be chaotic; it might be an immaculate and stylish penthouse apartment, a comfortable suburban house, or a squalid trailer in a mobile home park, but it is where we feel most comfortable. Comedian George Carlin said that home is where our stuff is. But it is also where we usually stuff the other important aspects of our lives: our mementos, our relationships, our most precious others. Maybe this isn't saying anything more than the sampler embroidered with "Home Is Where the Heart Is," but it's still true. And for most of us, it is also where we want our hearts to stop.

In addition to place, a good death also involves time. As I noted above, for some people, that desired time may be measured in seconds, but studies of those who are close to the end of their lives, as well as those who are recently bereaved, show that time is needed to die well, because there are things that need to be done. Some of these, like estate planning or choosing a funeral director, are simple check-off items, tasks that could be performed at any time, but the most important tasks possess and possibly require the urgency of an impending deadline.

A vital aspect of good death is the closing of relationships. Dr. Ira Byock, in his seminal work, *Dying Well*,[1] names "five things of relationship completion." These are tasks identified as five messages that almost every dying person needs to convey in order to achieve a healthy completion of their lives:

"Forgive me."
"I forgive you."
"Thank you."
"I love you."
"Good-bye."

As you contemplate those five statements and imagine the people you would need to say them to, as well as the emotional energy it would require to have those conversations, you can clearly see that these tasks are simple but not easy. Of course, we would all probably have healthier and happier lives if we didn't wait until the end to say some of those things; few of us get around to these important things while we are living day to day, assuming tomorrow. Many of my patients, as they approached their deaths, told me in one way or another that learning how to die taught them how to live.

It is obvious that the ones who know the most about what is important at the end of life, what makes for a good death, are those who are dying. But it has only been within the past couple of decades that anyone bothered to ask them about it. In a fascinating report published in 2000,[2] seriously ill patients, recently bereaved family members, physicians, and other care professionals (nurses, social workers, chaplains, and hospice volunteers) reported what they thought was most important at the end of life. There was some variation among the three groups surveyed. Pain relief, for example, was rated as important slightly more often by the physicians and care providers than it was by the patients, and maintaining a sense of humor, important to 93 percent of the patients, was way down the list for the doctors.

I have had many opportunities to speak with groups regarding the care of people at the end of life, and I have often used this study as a group exercise with a very loose *Family Feud*–type format, asking participants to guess the top five answers given by the patients. Most groups will get three or four of these, but only once did anyone come up with the top "survey says" response. Take a minute and think about it, then see how your guesses compare with the findings.

The number-five answer was to "have someone who will listen." Over and over, my patients told me how the health care system treated them like a number, a case, or a disease and never bothered to recognize them as individuals with hopes but mainly with fears. When they tried to talk with their neighbors and friends, these well-meaning folks were interested in the gory details about their disease, treatments, and doctors, but when they tried to communicate what they were really feeling, the conversation topic immediately changed, often to stories about somebody else who had something maybe like what they were dying from. Family members, and even clergy, were quick with advice, telling them what they should do without even asking what their big questions really were. And to talk with anyone about the fact that they were dying led to an abrupt "now don't talk like that, you need to keep a positive attitude" or a suddenly remembered obligation somewhere else. (As an aside here, if you ever wonder what you can do for someone who is seriously ill, dying, or recently bereaved, this is your clue: stop, keep quiet, take the time, and listen. The bumper sticker wisdom here is "don't just do something, sit there." It is of immense value.)

Number four on the list was to "know what to expect about one's physical condition." In the twenty years since this study was released there has been an explosion in the publication of patient information materials and decision-making aids. If you have undergone any significant medical procedure recently you have probably encountered these—a pamphlet handed to you at a doctor's office or maybe an online video for you to watch. These can be great for providing information about what happens during, say, a colonoscopy or cardiac bypass. Most hospice agencies also distribute materials to patients and families that describe common things that happen as the body weakens and organs shut down. Family members are reassured when the patient's symptoms are listed in the pamphlet. But sometimes the question the patient has is not in the book and not covered in the video. It is all too common for a doctor or nurse, after asking a patient, "Do you have any questions for me?" to feel irritated if they actually do, especially if that question is loaded with apprehension or fear. As a result, many patients and family members resort to online chat rooms and support groups on social media platforms as the default source of the information they want.

When there were doctors in my audience, I would often get a little dig in when we got to response number three: to "have a nurse with whom one feels comfortable." (Being able to trust one's doctor came in at number seven.) The patient's relationship with a nurse, particularly if it is long-standing, tends to be a more personal one than that with the physician, if only for the simple reason of time spent face to face. Patients and families see the nurse as one who has the necessary education and experience and who also has the priority of caring (maybe as opposed to curing). Cancer patients often develop trust and rapport with the chemotherapy nurses; in my oncology practice, patients would often bring in cookies, candy, or other treats, maybe handing them to me, but I knew they were really for the nurses. The nurse is the one with knowledge of what is likely to happen and who is more likely to be willing to listen, exactly what we've already seen as essential.

The second most commonly listed factor of importance at the end of life is the ability to "name a decision maker." We will discuss advance directives, the formal legal mechanisms to make sure that preferences are understood and carried out, in the next chapter, and those are very important. But there is more to this than just filling out a piece of paper. Honest reflection in selecting a surrogate decision maker and open conversations with that person can both increase the likelihood that one's wishes will be carried out and provide a sense of comfort that one has an advocate no matter what happens.

So, you ask, what factor was listed most often as important at the end of life? What was the "number-one answer"? It's not pain control, spiritual comfort, presence of family, or saying good-bye. It is to "be kept clean." I used this exercise with many groups, and the response when this answer was revealed was always "of course!" We don't want to die needing a bath, with repellent breath, sitting in our own dirty diaper. This is so obvious that, unless we are the one going through it, we don't even think about it. And that is the point I take away from this study; if we are going to provide better care for the dying, if we want to have a good death ourselves, we need to spend time learning about death and dying and what they might mean for us.

LILLIAN

I knew Lillian would be dead soon. She had come to our hospice unit from a local hospital where she had been treated for sepsis. She had colon cancer that had spread throughout her abdominal cavity and to her liver and lungs. Her primary need was to be rid of the constant nausea, repeated vomiting, and lancinating pain she was experiencing. Thanks to the medications we had started the day before, she felt like eating a little sausage and eggs that morning. But a couple hours later, the retching and pain recurred, this time accompanied by profuse bleeding from her rectum.

Her closest relative, a daughter-in-law, called to ask how she was doing. She said that no one at the hospital had told Lillian or her family just how bad her cancer was nor what to expect. It was clear to me that there was a disaster brewing in her abdomen—an obstructed, perforated, or even gangrenous intestine along with a bleeding tumor—and that this would cause her death in a very few days at most. We would most likely be able to manage most of her physical symptoms; there are effective medications and interventions to relieve the pain and vomiting that plague someone dying from bowel obstruction or peritonitis. But I needed to let Lillian in on just what was happening, what to expect.

Did she have to know? The hospice staff told me that during the times when her symptoms were less severe, she did not show signs of fear, anxiety, or emotional distress. I wondered if that meant she was not anxious or maybe just exhausted. I, along with virtually all who care for the dying, am convinced that people make better decisions, find their way more clearly, and finish their lives more comfortably if they understand the situation and know what they are up against. I was angry. Why hadn't the doctors at the hospital, or those who had treated her cancer for the past two years, told her what was happening? Or maybe they had provided

the facts, but Lillian and her family had not heard or compre-
hended the information. Miscommunication is endemic in the
medical system, after all. And now I was going to interrupt one of
her times of rest by giving her the news that all of us dread, that
she was dying, and that it would happen imminently.

Lillian was lying slightly propped up in her bed at the hospice
inpatient unit, tension evident in her muscles as she strained to
avoid any unnecessary movement. Even minor changes in body
position or movement of her legs produced piercing pain in her
abdomen. She weakly and mumblingly sang along with the gospel
music from the bedside CD player. Though she was clearly uncomfortable, when I entered the room she made sure to invite me
to pull the chair up next to her bed, her tastefully styled silver wig
only slightly askew, the sunlight from the window reflecting off the
stainless-steel cover over her uneaten lunch on the bedside table.

I deliver bad news all the time as part of my job. The steps have
become habit but are never routine. I know about getting the
setting right, asking what the patient already knows, delivering the
news, expecting the emotional response, and then summarizing,
establishing a plan, and giving reassurance. The emotional response is the unpredictable step; it is difficult to guess how people
will react. As she lay there, her dark brown skin and white teeth
set off by the jaundiced yellow discoloration in her eyes and the
red and purple of her bed jacket, I wondered about her response.
Would she cry or wail? Would she sniffle quietly and say nothing?
Would she try to relieve my suffering as so many do in this situation, saying, "Oh, Doctor, it must be so hard for you to have to do
this."

As I sat by her bedside, leaning forward, touching her hand, I
had second thoughts, wondering if I was just adding unnecessary
suffering; after all, she would likely be unconscious within not too
many hours as her body rapidly failed. But I said it: "Miss Lillian,
it looks like in the next few days you'll be going to heaven."

The relief of her tension was instantaneous. Her face brightened as she moved forward a bit and gleamingly said, "Oh, Doctor, that's the best thing you could have told me!" A few minutes

before she had winced at even the thought of movement, but now she leaned on her elbows, sitting up without even a grimace. I am certain the pain sensors in her abdomen were firing wildly, but at that moment her brain wasn't getting the message.

Lillian lived nearly a week after that, though she was unaware for most of it. During her times of lucidity, she prayed, and she thanked and blessed each one who examined her, gave her medications, and bathed her soiled body. She died the way she had lived; she died well.

DO AMERICANS GET GOOD DEATHS?

We noted above that the majority of Americans say that they want to die at home. But the most recent data show that no more than a third actually do so; the remainder of deaths occur about equally in hospitals and nursing homes.[3] For a large number of the elderly and disabled, a nursing home or assisted living facility becomes home, and increasing numbers of those organizations exhibit interest and care to improve the way people die in their institutions, making a good death more possible.

The big disconnect, though, is in the hospital setting, where at least a quarter of all deaths occur. It is here that the good death, the death many imagine for themselves, is most difficult to achieve. In order to sort through this disconnect, we need to review some of what happened in medical care over the past century. Up until the antibiotic era (Sir Alexander Fleming discovered penicillin in 1928), the leading cause of death was infectious diseases such as pneumonia and gangrene, which killed quickly, and tuberculosis and syphilis, which took their time. Death occurred to people of all ages; an infant was nearly as likely to die as a grandmother. The dying process was a familiar one; everyone had firsthand experience of losing someone they knew, a parent, child, or sibling. It was just a part of life. People died at home; there was nowhere else to go. Family members provided all the hands-on care, unless they could afford servants to do the dirty work.

As wonder drugs and surgical advances began to cure more and more previously fatal conditions, the picture changed. Dying might be avoided or at least put off. Mortality statistics did change; dying increasingly became something that might not happen until one reached an advanced age. But to beat the grim reaper, one had to get the best medicine when one got sick. Hospitals became places for curing disease, so that's where sick people went to get better. Medical technology could now step in when organs failed: ventilators keep people breathing, dialysis machines replace failed kidneys, intravenous feeding keep the nutrition flowing. All these interventions were done with the idea that if the patient could be kept going, the doctors would eventually find the right treatment to fix all the problems. Hospitals even began to advertise themselves as having particular expertise in curing disease, preventing death. This attitude is most evident today on health system billboards, in television and print media ads, and in the importance placed on U.S. News and World Report rankings. Sometimes this death-defying attitude took a hubristic tone, with more than one hospital administrator or physician chief of staff being heard to say, "Patients do not die here." Of course, people did and do die in hospitals, those denials notwithstanding. The same year that the chief of staff of our hospital made that claim, funeral directors made some seven hundred visits there to pick up corpses.

Dying in the hospital wasn't pretty. In the early 1990s, the Study to Understand Prognoses and Preferences for Outcomes and Risks of Treatments (SUPPORT) showed that seriously ill patients, with a predictable and high likelihood of dying, spent their last days in the intensive care unit, receiving mechanical ventilation, in moderate to severe pain, or, if they were lucky, comatose.[4] This pattern is aptly described by Dr. Jessica Nutik Zitter in her book *Extreme Measures* as "The End of Life Conveyor Belt."[5] The doctors and hospital staff who were part of the SUPPORT study recognized that these results were unacceptable, and many expressed a powerful desire to improve. What was disheartening, though, was the follow-up study, in which trained nurses met with patients and families to determine their understanding and preferences, then communicated this information to the doctors and nurses taking care of the patient, sometimes facilitating family meetings with the medical staff. Even with motivated clinicians and this much-improved communication, the outcomes did not improve. Dying patients continued to suffer and be subjected to futile procedures. Doctors and hospitals kept trying to cure even when they knew it couldn't succeed because that's what they knew how to do; there just did not seem to be another option. The high-technology, disease-fighting paradigm that was so successful in curing illness and saving lives, the same medical care system responsible for all those apparent miracles, systematically failed when it came to caring for those whose illnesses could not be cured, whose lives could not be saved.

Fortunately, over the past two decades, doctors, hospitals, health care systems, and regulations have made significant improvements, especially in pain control and documenting advance directives. Pain became the "fifth vital sign," and now, whenever someone encounters the medical system, they are asked if they are having any pain and, if so, to rate it on a scale from one to ten. In 1990, Congress passed the Patient Self-Determination Act, requiring that all hospitals and nursing homes that receive federal funding (and since this includes Medicare and Medicaid, the rule is virtually universal) provide patients an opportunity to complete a living will and durable power of attorney for health care. Financial and regulatory pressures altered the whole dynamic of acute hospitalization and shifted much care to the outpatient setting. The voices of patients, especially autonomy-valuing baby boomers, pushed for more and earlier conversations and decisions. These forces, as well as the growth of hospices and palliative care programs, have clarified other available options. When I served as director of the palliative care program at a large university hospital, I thought that a significant value we provided was that we "gave structure to the 'or.'" Patients and families were, and unfortunately too often still are, asked, "So do you want us to keep doing everything, or . . ." Without knowing what that "or" looks like, how could anyone recommend or choose it?

Things are changing. In 2000, about 33 percent of Medicare patients who died did so in the hospital; by 2009 this was down to 25 percent.[6] Those who received hospice care (discussed in chapter 3) increased from 22 percent to 42 percent. But during that same time, the number who had been in the intensive care unit during the last month of their life increased from 24 percent to 29 percent. These numbers are open to several possible interpretations. Does aggressive care extend life or prolong dying? Are patients given more good quality time or robbed of it? These are difficult questions, and there are no easy answers.

One thing we know, though, is that the aggressive disease-oriented approach comes with a cost. Most patients I cared for who were transferred from a hospital to our hospice inpatient unit reported that while they were hospitalized their personal needs and questions were seldom satisfied. They acknowledged that the doctors and hospital staff had been honest and respectful in communicating what was wrong and that they were dying (a significant improvement!), but once the focus became comfort rather than cure, the doctors, in particular, seemed less interested in them. There are many otherwise good doctors who, because of lack of interest or training, don't see these patients as those they can "do" anything more for and so cede control to social workers, nurses, and discharge planners. I was personally taken aback when one physician, who frequently referred elderly nursing home patients to our hospice agency, said that "once the patient is on hospice, it becomes boring." I must somehow admire this doctor's honesty in recognizing how he felt and articulating it, but so many of my patients who had experiences like this told me that they felt abandoned.

Much has changed in the century and a half since the Civil War and even since 1939, the year *Gone with the Wind* won the Oscar for Best Picture, but people still die and always will. For some, life is extinguished in an unsuspecting moment; others receive the gift of advance warning and opportunity for life resolution. If we want to ensure, as best we can, that our own dying occurs in a way consistent with our lives and values, we must acknowledge the reality of our own mortality, contemplate our values and wishes for that time, and make reasonable preparations. In the next chapter, we will look at the tools available to make sure that our wishes are carried out.

2

I'M GOING TO DIE? WHAT CAN I DO?

Dying is only bad when it takes a long time and hurts so much that it humiliates you.
—Ernest Hemingway, *For Whom the Bell Tolls*

Dorothy didn't have cancer after all, but she died anyway. She was a portly woman, well into her eighties, with white hair, a gravelly voice, and a crusty personality. I felt like I was being graded when I visited her, probably because she reminded me of my elementary school teachers. Dorothy was referred for hospice care with a diagnosis of metastatic cancer. She had undergone an evaluation for abdominal pain, and this showed a fluid-filled growth in her pelvis and a two-inch mass in her liver. Her doctor told her that there was no way that this was not cancer, and Dorothy decided that she was done with tests and procedures, so a biopsy was never done. She said that she did not want to be told any more bad news; the information that she was dying of cancer was enough. She decided to just live the remainder of her life the best she could.

But she didn't die. She didn't even lose weight, like people with advanced cancers do. And her appetite, especially for Hershey bars and ice cream, remained excellent. She continued receiving hospice care; that's what she wanted. Her aches and pains, shortness of breath, and anxiety had never been controlled as well as we had been able to do. But now it was going on a year since she had been referred with a diagnosis that should have caused major problems, if not her death, by this time.

DEATH IS PERSONAL

In the time that it took you to read this much of Dorothy's story, five Americans died. In 2017, there were 2,813,503 deaths in the United States.[1] About a quarter of Americans die of heart disease, some 22 percent from cancer, and about one in twenty each for stroke and accidents. But there is one statistic that doesn't get included in CDC reports: the overall risk of dying, which is, of course, 100 percent. The most common cause of death is being alive. We all know this. We intellectually acknowledge that our lives are not permanent. Most people feel uncomfortable thinking, let alone talking, about their own death. When I have conversations with patients and families, people often say things like, "I mean, I know everybody is going to die . . ." often followed with a half laugh and a "but . . ." What I heard when people said this was, "Everybody is going to die . . . except me." We think of ourselves as exceptional. When I see a car veer all over the road, with the driver texting behind the wheel, I imagine that if I challenged the driver as to why they were doing it, I would be told that they are an excellent driver, good at multitasking, don't really do it that often, or some other excuse. These rationalizations would imply that they know the rules and the dangers of texting and driving but see them as irrelevant to their own behavior. Maybe you don't text and drive; maybe you rationalize speeding, eating too much, smoking, ignoring weather alerts, or cheating on your spouse or your income tax. We try to justify our behavior despite the known potential consequences; we seem to think that we will be the one who gets away with it. If we can deny these personal risks, even as we find ourselves halfway off the road, needing to buy larger pants, or called in for an audit, how much easier is it to avoid the personal reality of dying, an event we assume will be far in the future?

Harvard physician and end-of-life researcher Susan Block wrote, "Arriving at an acceptance of one's mortality and a clear understanding of the limits and the possibilities of medicine is a process, not an epiphany."[2] One advantage of recognizing the personal inevitability of your own death is that when the time comes, the idea will be neither novel nor shocking. You will have already done some of the inner screaming and weeping and will be just a bit more prepared to make the decisions and do the work required of you.

None of us remember the moment of our birth, but we all know we went through it; there is just no other way of getting here. It is almost unimaginable to think of ourselves as slimy, wrinkled infants, but we've seen the pictures and have heard the stories from our parents. Since your birth likely seems unreal to you, take a moment, maybe the next time you step out of the bath or shower, and look at your navel in the mirror. It may be an innie or an outie, it may be pierced and sexy or hiding between abdominal folds, but it is there. It is a durable reminder that you were once a fetus being kept alive through that button in your belly. That wrinkled dimple is lasting proof that you joined with every other member of the human race in being born. And as such, it is also permanent evidence that you will die. Nobody gets out of here alive.

I know this very well. I am a doctor whose patients all died. I am a hospice physician; all my patients have been told they will die in the next several months, most even sooner. I didn't start out in medicine that way, though. When I completed my training in hematology and medical oncology, full of scientific facts and wet-behind-the-ears enthusiasm, I was ready to take on complex diagnostic dilemmas and cure cancers. I knew that disease was the enemy and that my commission was to take the fight to that foe. It didn't take me long to realize, though, that rules of engagement were considerably less clear on the front lines than they were in the textbooks, journals, and conferences.

My patients, like all patients of all doctors, wanted me to be aggressive, to fight for them, and I did that with all the skill and armaments at my disposal. But there is something fundamentally flawed in this commonly held militaristic view of cancer treatment. The battlefield where the war is waged is not the cancer cell, the CT scan results, or the blood counts; rather it is the body of a human being, a body belonging to a person with fears, hopes, dreams, and nightmares. Whether or not the treatment works against the disease, the patient gets the side effects. Unfortunately, a few oncologists cope with the reality of disease, the adverse effects of treatment, and the deterioration and death they see every day by "hating cancer more than they like people." Every doctor that treats patients with high-risk, life-threatening disease must find their own defense mechanisms to protect them from the suffering and dying they see so often. I suspect that this is part of what engendered the intensive care unit culture that was identified by the SUPPORT study and eloquently described by Dr. Zitter, as mentioned in the previous chapter.

My coping strategy evolved in a different direction. I discovered a personal interest in those who walked into my office, lay on my examination tables, sat for interminable intravenous infusions, and went home knowing they would be throwing up a few hours later. It was the relationships with these people I encountered each day that got me up every morning and gave meaning to my practice. This was true (mostly) even for the times when the names of those I dreaded to see were on my schedule. I treated cancer aggressively—after all, that's what they came to me for, to fight their disease—but, when they would allow, I also shared a bit of their lives and revealed a bit of mine. Births, marriages, grandchildren, graduations, job losses, crop production, and the county fair were frequent topics of discussion, along with the nausea and vomiting, hair loss, low blood counts, and results of the latest scans.

In Wooster, Ohio, where I practiced, a small not-for-profit hospice agency relied on local physicians, clergy, and many other volunteers to supplement the skills and dedication of their employed staff. It was through this work with Hospice of Wayne County, in making home visits when needed, that I learned the immeasurable value of presence. By continuing to care for my cancer patients until they died, I acquired insight into the equally essential virtue of nonabandonment. When I first attended a hospice and palliative medicine conference in the early 1990s, I realized that I had found my home—a community of professionals of various disciplines who had found what I had discovered: that it is the people, not the diseases, that matter. It would be years before I would totally focus my medical practice on the care of the dying, but in the meantime, the lessons I learned from those at the end of their lives made me a better oncologist and maybe even a better person. As I mentioned above, the most important of those lessons is the realization that I also am mortal, and I too will die.

DOROTHY

I talked with Dorothy about whether there might have been a mistake in her original diagnosis. She asked, "You mean I might not really have cancer?" When she heard she was dying, she had changed her lifestyle, moving to an expensive assisted living facility. But now, after more than a year, her money had run out and she had to go on Medicaid and enter a nursing home. She had adjusted to the idea of being terminally ill and was resistant to abandoning that self-image and losing the benefits that came with it. She dreaded giving up her hospice team, though we assured her that the nursing home staff could do an excellent job in managing her symptom medicines. For Dorothy, though, it wasn't the drugs that were most important. Her gruff demeanor had distanced her from her family; it was the members of her hospice team who had been consistently with her through these past months. I reviewed with her that one of my responsibilities as a hospice medical director was to confirm that she was terminally ill. Since her body had not shown any evidence of deterioration, I needed some new medical information to be able to reaffirm that hospice care remained appropriate for her. She reluctantly agreed to an abdominal ultrasound to see just what was happening with this cancer she had been told would kill her.

The ultrasound showed no mass in her liver, just some minor chronic gallbladder disease. She never had cancer. About a week before Christmas, we met with her at the nursing home to give her the good news. The tears that welled up in her eyes, that streamed down her cheeks, testified both to the fact that she would miss the hospice nurses and aides that she had come to know and to the joy she felt from her new lease on life, her resurrection. And it was my joy to plant a brief kiss on the moist cheek of this crusty old woman as I said good-bye.

ADVANCE CARE PLANNING

If you watch much late night or cable television, you will have seen the commercials for the various "final expense" insurance plans promoted by numerous companies. They emphasize the financial cost of funerals and recommend planning for these expenses, using their product, of course. Whether these promoted services are the best financial plan can be debated, but the advertisements are correct when they suggest that if we want some control over the circumstances of our dying, we need to plan for it.

Advance care planning is the process of communicating preferences regarding future health care needs should one become unable to speak for oneself. This can be informal, such as having a talk with your family over Thanksgiving dinner, or more formalized, enacting legal documents to specify your preferences or name the person you want to speak for you. These formal processes are called advance directives.

Advance Directives

As a result of high-profile court cases starting in the mid-1970s, the idea of advance directives became a popular concept. State legislatures have enacted statutes establishing the legal basis for these directives and their enforcement, and courts have consistently upheld them. The underlying concept is based on the principle of autonomy, that a competent adult has the right to accept or refuse virtually any medical treatment or intervention. If you have had a medical procedure performed, you've signed an "informed consent" form indicating that you understand what is proposed, what the risks and benefits are, and agree to it being done—that is, you agree to undergo the proposed treatment. An advance directive is similar in that it anticipates common scenarios involving terminal illness and provides your consent or refusal of specific medical interventions in those cases, should you be unable to speak for yourself.

While the specific details of advance directive rules vary from state to state, there are two types of documents that are accepted nationwide. (I use the term "document" because a written form or statement is the most common method of providing these instructions, though in many situations oral or other communication is allowed.) The first type of advance directive is the living will, a document that communicates your preferences for care if you are dying or in a persistent comatose state. Commonly, living wills direct refusal of resuscitation, intensive care, ventilators, and other aggressive support devices, and request measures to provide comfort. The use of artificial nutrition and hydration, sometimes called tube feeding, is also usually included, often as a separate statement. While a living will provides information on your choices and may be useful to family and caregivers, it only becomes enforceable in the situations it describes—that is, if you are terminally ill and unable to speak for yourself or in an irreversible coma. If, for example, you develop Alzheimer's disease and lose the ability to communicate but are not at the end of your life, it has no force. Often, doctors and hospitals will use the fact that a patient has a living will as evidence to suggest that they should not institute aggressive and intensive medical care, but there is no legal need for them to do so.

The other more flexible and commonly useful advance directive is the durable power of attorney for health care (DPAH). Using this tool, you give a specific person the authority to speak for you, to make medical decisions on your behalf, when you are unable to speak for yourself. The person you name as your DPAH can be an effective advocate in ensuring that the choices that are made are those you would make for yourself. To make the DPAH especially valuable, be sure you have communicated your desires with your designated surrogate, that they understand your values, hopes, and fears. There are a few legal restrictions to the full authority of a DPAH. For example, in many jurisdictions,* their authority to remove life-support machines is limited if you are not terminally ill or if you are pregnant.

If you do not name a DPAH, when guidance is needed, the doctors and hospital taking care of you will seek out someone to speak for you. Given the fact that less than a third of Americans have named someone as their agent, this is a common scenario. Unfortunately, state laws vary considerably as far as who can be named the legal surrogate for someone who does not name one themselves.[3] Some states have no statute at all. Many list relatives, ranking them in order of priority. Some states allow non-DPAH surrogacy only in matters of life and death but not in others, and statutes vary considerably as far as if and how surrogacy can be challenged. From a practical standpoint, especially in emergency situations, doctors will usually ask whatever family member is present to assist in making a decision. But remember that the point of having someone act as your spokesperson is for them to communicate what you would want to be done, not what they think should happen. It is in your best interest to be sure that the one who speaks for you is the one who knows what you would want and who is willing and able to advocate for that.

Let's look at how these work in the real world. I have a living will and DPAH document, naming my wife as my primary designated agent, and we live and receive our medical care in Ohio. My living will carries force of state law if I am in a terminal condition and unable to make my own health care decisions or if I am in a permanently unconscious state, both of which are defined in the statute. It directs my physician to administer no life-sustaining treatment, including CPR and artificially or technologically supplied nutrition and hydration, to withdraw any such treatment already started, to issue a "do not resuscitate" order, and to permit me to die naturally. It also says to take no action to postpone my death but to provide me with care necessary to make me comfortable and relieve my pain. This is fairly straightforward, but, as noted above, it comes into force only in the two specific situations it describes.

My DPAH states that my agent (my wife) has authority to make health care decisions for me if I cannot do so. It says that she will make those decisions based on any specific instructions I have included in the document as well as any other information and opinions that I have personally communicated to her. This gives her virtual authority to be my voice in giving or withdrawing consent to any medical procedure as well as any other related decision, like obtaining medical records, choosing a doctor, and transporting me to a facility that honors my DPAH if I am in a place that does not do so. There are a few specific things she cannot do: she can't kill me by refusing life-saving treatment if I am not otherwise terminally ill, and she can't make me suffer by refusing comfort medications for me.

The DPAH and living will are essential documents for ensuring that your wishes will be carried out if you cannot speak for yourself, but they have significant limitations. First, if a doctor or hospital is to adhere to your instructions, they must know that these documents exist. You should make sure that your doctor and any hospital you enter knows that you have executed these instructions and provide them with a copy. Hospitals are required to ask about them when you are admitted, so be sure that anyone who might transport you when you are ill knows that you have them. One of the goals of transition to electronic medical records, especially as envisioned by the Affordable Care Act, was to make records, including these advance directives, immediately available in electronic format wherever a patient presented themselves. But as of now, this is far from reality, and the political climate does not suggest that it will occur any time soon.

Another flaw in the implementation of advance directives is that, even with the content of the documents known, they still may not be followed. This is almost always done with the best of intentions. The most common problem is the unavailability of the designated spokesperson. Emergency personnel work hard to find and notify family of a critically ill patient. Doctors and nurses generally act to save and support life, so sometimes procedures get performed that the patient would not have desired. This is not an irreversible situation; DPAH and living will documents authorize the withdrawal of undesired treatment. From ethical and legal standpoints, in almost every situation, removing a treatment is treated as equivalent to never starting it in the first place.

More bothersome, though, are situations in which instructions are known, and the authorized surrogate is contacted, but the patient's desires are overruled. Fortunately, it is becoming rare for a physician to disparage the statements of a stressed family member DPAH with comments like "So, you just want us to let your mom die?" But guilt and conflict still can cause a surrogate to override the desired action, especially if there is underlying family conflict. A sibling with a more forceful personality, or maybe a long-standing domineering relationship with the one named as DPAH, can sometimes coerce others to get their own way. A particularly tricky situation for medical staff can occur if the designated spokesperson is only available by phone and another family member is present, confronting the staff, threatening legal action if their own wishes are not obeyed.

Advance directives are generally used to prevent someone from having to undergo undesired treatment—that is, they are used to ensure what might be called a negative right, the right to not have what you don't want. The only positive right supported by these documents is the right to receive treatment aimed at comfort and pain relief. It is, of course, possible to put other instructions in an advance directive, things you do want done, but enforcement might be problematic. Patients have the right to accept or refuse but not to demand a specific treatment or procedure. This is particularly relevant in the current situation in which certain medical procedures, such as medical marijuana, are allowed in some jurisdictions but not in others. In states that have legalized medical aid in dying, the patient must request this procedure personally; it cannot be obtained through advance directive or a DPAH. And with regard to organ donation, in most states, even though individuals' choice to be an organ donor is published on their driver's license, they cannot actually authorize the organ removal to occur. This final authority is given to the surviving next of kin after death has occurred.

Anticipatory Physician Orders: DNR and POLST

A final limitation of living wills and DPAH documents is that, although they carry the force of law, this does not include the authority of a doctor's order. My living will provides my directions to the physician caring for me, who then will initiate the orders that will carry out my wishes. A common exception occurs when the first to encounter a critically ill patient is the emergency medical technician. These experts in saving lives are charged to do so, and they generally require either a clearly futile situation (a body clearly dead, a decapitated corpse, etc.) or a physician's order to not proceed with resuscitation and life support. This has led to the idea, enacted in many jurisdictions, of "portable" prewritten directives that include an authorized doctor's order.

The most common of these is the portable do not resuscitate (DNR) form. This legal form, signed by your physician (and usually by you), says that in the event your heart stops, or if you stop breathing, that cardiopulmonary resuscitation (CPR) should not be started and that every effort should be made to ensure your comfort. The "portability" of the form is that it is in force in any site within the state of its execution. For my patients living at home, I recommend they put it on the front of the refrigerator or in some other prominent place so it will be seen by an ambulance crew. For a patient in a nursing home, this is kept in the chart, sometimes in the room also, and a copy goes with them if they are transferred to a hospital.

Avoiding attempts at emergency resuscitation is important for those with chronic serious illnesses. CPR and advanced cardiac life support (ACLS) were developed for people who suffer a sudden fatal heart rhythm abnormality, usually in the setting of a heart attack. This is also the point of the placement of automated defibrillators in public places. Televised medical dramas frequently portray resuscitation attempts, or "codes," and on TV they are successful most of the time. The real data, though, are quite different. For someone suffering a heart attack in public, with the initiation of bystander CPR, quick use of an automated defibrillator, and prompt arrival of an emergency medical team, the chances of making it to the hospital alive are 24 percent, but less than one in ten ever make it to hospital discharge.[4] The situation is much worse for someone with multiple chronic medical problems, in whom the success rates approach zero. In addition, many who do survive the resuscitation effort suffer significant brain or other organ damage from the lack of blood flow. The "code" procedure itself in chronically ill patients often results in rib fractures and other injuries.

In the past, patients in hospitals or nursing homes with DNR orders received inferior medical care, as if DNR somehow meant "do not treat." Currently, more and more physicians, hospitals, and extended care facilities recognize that DNR can just mean that the patient does not want to undergo a traumatic and ineffective procedure yet desires all other appropriate medical treatment. Some state regulations recognize this also. In Ohio, for example, the portable DNR statute provides two options: DNRCC (comfort care) that puts the focus on pain and symptom control and away from life-prolonging measures, and DNRCC-Arrest, which allows any medical treatment except CPR and the "code." Unfortunately, the way the differences are expressed and explained in the regulations and documents confuse rather than clarify exactly what is desired and ordered. A decision on a DNR order itself, while often emotionally difficult, is straightforward. But the usual pathway of chronic and progressive serious illness includes numerous other forks, decisions that need to be made.

As an example, consider that you are the named DPAH for your elderly mother, who has Alzheimer's disease and has recently been admitted to a nursing home. She has high blood pressure, type 2 diabetes, and chronic obstructive lung disease caused by smoking when she was younger. All these conditions have been well controlled by her current medicines. Her major problems, the ones that resulted in her inability to continue to care for herself, are her advanced age, frailty, and worsening dementia. You have had an open and honest relationship with your mother, and you feel confident in your understanding of her values, hopes, and fears. You know that she would not want to go through CPR, be put on breathing machines, or have a feeding tube inserted if she lost the ability to swallow. As such, establishing a DNR is an easy decision.

But little old ladies with dementia don't usually just drop dead. What do you do if she breaks her hip? She has been able to walk around fairly well using a cane, but her only chance to resume doing that will require hip surgery followed by weeks of physical therapy and rehabilitation that she may not be able to cooperate with or even endure. So, do you send her to the hospital in the hope she might walk again, or do you avoid surgery, request increased pain medicine, and keep her mainly in bed, hoping that, if she survives the acute episode and when the pain from the acute injury calms down, she will eventually be able to transfer into a wheelchair to get around? Or, as in a different and even more common scenario, if she gets pneumonia and has trouble breathing do you send her to the hospital, do you ask for antibiotic pills at the nursing home, or do you request only interventions to lessen her shortness of breath, knowing that if she dies, well, pneumonia used to be called the "old person's friend"?

There have been attempts to develop advance directives that try to anticipate potential medical problems and complications and decide what you would desire done in those situations. The most common of these approaches are termed Physician Orders for Life Sustaining Treatment (POLST).[5] The concept is the same as the portable DNR, but here the scope is expanded. Choices can be made for artificial feeding, antibiotics, hospitalization, intravenous fluids, and other specific medical interventions. As we have discovered, one problem is that it is difficult to envision every scenario that might be encountered and that you might choose differently depending on the nuances of the situation. But, particularly for those with advanced diseases or dementia, nearing the end of their lives, POLST can establish their desires in writing, and, in states with corresponding statutes, with the force of physician order and legal enforceability.

While advance directive legislation and policies are ubiquitous, and numerous states have established POLST programs, they have not always changed the way Americans experience medical care at the end of their life. This is because there are just too many holes in the way information is communicated and decisions are implemented. A well-intentioned nurse on temporary night duty at an unfamiliar assisted living facility finds a resident struggling to breathe and calls 911. The responding emergency medical technicians initiate oxygen and other treatment and quickly transport to the local hospital emergency department, where the triage nurse identifies the patient as critically ill and the emergency physician diagnoses pneumonia and initiates antibiotics and admission to the intensive care unit. There the intensivist uses the medical marvels at hand to support and try to save the patient. This common scenario, an example of the superb system we have in this country to cure disease and save lives, involves at least five transition points, transfers of care of the patient from one person or setting to another. Each of these transfers requires effective communication but also provides the opportunity for someone to "press pause" and to ask if this is what the patient wants done. Unfortunately, it is at these points of transition of care that the greatest likelihood for error and missed opportunities occur.

Some jurisdictions and health systems are starting to address the complexities inherent in care transitions and decision making. The state of Oregon is a leader here, with efforts to educate professionals and the public as well as changes in state EMS and Medical Board regulations. The result is that persons dying in that state are less likely to be hospitalized and more likely to use hospice services than those in the rest of the country.[6] This demonstrates that thoughtful systemic changes can result in improvements in practice and patient care. The firestorm that surrounds issues of health care at the federal level, though, indicates that the chances of those types of changes being implemented on a national scale are remote. In the meantime, then, for the highest likelihood of your wishes being carried out, you should not only execute advance directive documents but also communicate their presence, location, and content to your family, friends, and care providers. In short, prospectively advocate for yourself and your wishes. A living will form lying in a file drawer with your other estate documents might get noticed, but most likely only when you are dead, and then it is too late.

Food and Water

In the discussion above, we encountered the issue of what is termed "artificial nutrition and hydration" (ANH). In typical living will forms, this is often put in a separate section that requires specific authorization by the person executing the living will. This is because not all people, including ethicists, politicians, and religious leaders, agree on whether this should be considered an "extraordinary" medical procedure or the more "ordinary" provision of basic human needs.

ANH can take many forms, but the prototypical method is the placement of a feeding tube into the stomach or small intestine of the patient. This is most commonly done using the technique of percutaneous endoscopic gastrostomy (PEG). In this procedure, a doctor inserts an endoscope (a black, flexible, lighted tube like the one so familiar to all of us middle-aged Americans who get cancer screenings) through the mouth and esophagus into the stomach, identifying the best site for insertion of a feeding tube through the abdominal wall into the stomach, where it is secured in place. The PEG provides permanent access through which a patient can then receive nutrition, hydration, and medications. The feedings can be thinly puréed "normal" food but more often consist of commercial nutritional products, similar to baby formula but designed for adults. A PEG can be lifesaving for the patient with injury of the mouth or throat, or cancer of the esophagus, or a myriad of other conditions that interfere with the body's ability to eat and swallow.

So, what is the problem? Well, let's suppose you suffer from esophageal cancer. Your PEG has been a boon to getting through treatment and living a fulfilling life, but now the cancer has recurred and is growing despite treatment. Is the nutrition, delivered through the PEG, keeping up your strength and quality of life or is it just prolonging the duration of your suffering? If ANH is a medical procedure, then stopping it is no different than discontinuing hemodialysis, chemotherapy, or a breathing machine. But if ANH equals eating and drinking, then stopping it could be seen as intentionally starving to death, committing suicide.

So, we need some perspective and some facts. In virtually every society, eating and drinking are not just biological functions; they are social events. Mother and infant bond as the baby nurses. Toddlers celebrate their birthday by eating cake and ice cream with their playmates. Adolescents make their first steps into relationships over burgers or pizza. Families mark joyous and sorrowful occasions with meals together. Leaders of nations forge alliances at state dinners. Grandparents make cookies for their grandchildren. And occasionally those grandchildren later get to give that grandparent a few small spoonfuls of ice cream as a final, loving gesture.

But administration of ANH is more like giving a dose than eating a meal. A common process is for a bag full of nutrients to be hooked up each evening, with the contents slowly infused overnight using a pump device that looks very much like the familiar IV pumps we've all seen in hospitals. Even the words "nutrition and hydration" as opposed to "food and drink" connote a more biological than cultural meaning. From a legal standpoint, in 1990 the US Supreme Court ruled, in the case of Nancy Cruzan (discussed further in chapter 5), that there is no difference between ANH and a mechanical ventilator as far as both are life-sustaining technologies. This decision placed ANH in the realm of "extraordinary" medical procedures. As discussed earlier in this chapter, though, some religious or ethical authorities maintain opinions that differ from this finding. And when the administration of a health care facility, like a nursing home, adheres to those differing opinions, it can impinge on your right to act on your desires. Administrators have no authority to tell a patient that they cannot stop their tube feeding, but they may well have the authority to say that you cannot stop tube feeding while remaining a resident in that facility.

A particularly troubling epidemic developed in the 1990s in the care of persons with advanced Alzheimer's disease and other dementias. One frequent complication of dementia is the loss of the ability to eat—first, of course, losing the ability to feed oneself, then having a progressively difficult time swallowing, resulting in food or fluid "going down the wrong way," entering the trachea and lungs (called aspiration) instead of the esophagus and stomach. This raises the risk of aspiration pneumonia, a serious lung infection. The risk of aspiration can be lessened by careful attention to swallowing techniques, but for many patients with dementia, this is an impossible task. An alternative, since thin liquids are more likely to be aspirated than thicker material, is a change in diet, switching to puréed food and thickened liquids. Again, this can help, but it decreases the pleasure of eating (have you ever tried thickened water?). But often the eventual result was the determination that the patient had a high risk for aspirating over and over again and getting repeated pneumonia. So, the solution was the PEG tube. If they don't swallow, they can't aspirate, right?

It became common practice for a patient, after, say, hospitalization for pneumonia to be discharged to the nursing home (even if they hadn't been there before—after all, they've got a new medical device the family isn't sure about) with a new tube in their stomach and a prescription for tube feedings.

The problem is, it doesn't work. A review published in 1999 documented that tube feeding in patients with advanced dementia does not prevent aspiration pneumonia and does little to protect against complications of malnutrition, like bedsores, other infections, and weakness.[7] There is also no evidence that PEG feeding in these patients allows them to live longer. But the story gets worse, because tube feeding results in complications from the tube, the procedure to put it in, and the need to sedate or restrain the patient to keep them from pulling the tube out. And the volume of material being pumped into the stomach can actually increase the risk that some will migrate up the esophagus and down into the lungs. Fortunately, this knee-jerk approach to swallowing difficulty in elderly demented patients is becoming less frequent, but it persists.

An effective alternative is careful, slow hand feeding by caring trained family members or staff. This takes time and costs money for care facilities—one reason tube feedings caught on so quickly. Skilled and slow hand feeding while reminding the patient to swallow can achieve what PEG feeding does not.

But sometimes a patient does not want even this. My friend Joseph confided in me the struggles he was having achieving the kind of life's end that his mother, Madeline, had told him she wanted. Madeline was a voraciously independent woman, and she had no desire to linger in an undignified state. She became an early member of the organization then known as the Hemlock Society, a group committed to the right of individuals to end their lives, with medical assistance if possible (medical aid in dying, discussed in chapter 4), when the burdens of ongoing life and suffering were unbearable. Madeline executed specific advance directives and named Joseph as her DPAH. She included instruction not only that she not have ANH but also that, should she get to the point at which she was unable to feed herself and was unable to interact or function as a person, she not be given food or water at all so that her life could end more quickly.

Madeline's body remained healthy, but she developed dementia that worsened to the point that she was bedfast, incontinent, noncommunicative, and unable to eat. She was losing weight and weakening. It was clear that she was dying. Hospice care was instituted. Joseph met with the administration and care staff of the excellent facility where his mother was living and advocated for what his mother had demanded of him, that she not be given any food or liquids. It took several conversations; nursing homes, after all, are graded based on the support they provide their residents, and one of those supports is nutrition. Also, the idea of "comfort feeding," bites and sips for flavor if nothing else, is usually viewed as an enhancement of quality of life.

Joseph became irritated, then angry, when he found that one of the nursing assistants, a gentle and caring woman named Lucita, had been surreptitiously slipping Madeline nibbles of ice cream and small syringes of water. He insisted that this be stopped but did not want to cost this compassionate caregiver her job. Lucita was transferred to another wing, Madeline died peacefully, and Joseph knew he had acted honorably but still wrestled with the whole experience.

Joseph wanted me to tell his mother's story as an example of how difficult it can be to ensure that one's advance directives are followed. He believes that his mother suffered by being subjected to something she did not want and by possibly having her life extended and that Lucita was in the wrong in her duplicitous but well-meaning actions. Bioethicists are divided on the correct action in this situation. Clearly, Madeline, in her pre-dementia, whole-person state, would have agreed that the tastes of ice cream were a violation of her wishes and bodily integrity. But was that the person that Lucita encountered? Is the dying patient with dementia the same person with the same values as the prior version of themselves? Perhaps Lucita could only see the woman in front of her, a pathetic but human creature whose sole awareness was that she was hungry.

Lucita was reprimanded and reassigned. Joseph continues to hold that her actions were wrong and that his mother's previously strongly stated wishes were the paramount value. I'm not so sure what the correct answer is. I strongly value both personal autonomy and relief of suffering. Sometimes it's just complicated.

☼ ☼ ☼

My peck on Dorothy's cheek didn't turn out to be good-bye. Maybe it was excitement from finding out she wasn't going to die, less likely the surprise kiss from her doctor, but only a few hours later the stroke struck. She lost the use of her left side, her ability to swallow, and most of her communication capability. When I saw her the next day, she stared without focus up and over my shoulder, trying to plead, "Help me." Her heart had gone into an abnormal rhythm, and a blood clot had formed in her left atrium and had traveled to her brain. Within two days she was dead.

BIRTH, DEATH, LIVING

When I was born, in the 1950s, most of us entered the world under the glare of surgical lights, our mothers drugged, our fathers absent. Birth was viewed as a medical procedure. Thanks particularly to women for whom this was unacceptable, giving birth is now seen as a natural process, best directed by the people actually doing it—the mothers. The purpose of medical personnel and facilities are assistance and safety. After all, being born is just a part of what we call life, full of blood and beauty, pain and wonder.

As we have seen, dying is now also treated as a medical event, often accompanied by lights, machines, monitors, tubes, and isolation. Sometimes this is just the way it has to be. We did not choose the moment or method of our birth and, even with advance directives and the best of intentions, we are not guaranteed the ability to choose the circumstances of our death. Sometimes a heart attack, a drunk driver, a flawed communication system, or an insistent family member takes our choice away.

But the main point is not really about the dying itself, is it? It is really about living, living that last part of our lives as well as or better than we've lived the rest of it. We have seen that a good death usually includes planning, effort, and time. Advance directives are usually used to say what we don't want, but what about what we do want? The next chapter will look at resources available to help us in living this last part of our lives.

3

HOSPICE

You matter because you are you, and you matter to the last moment of your life. We will do all we can, not only to help you die peacefully, but to live until you die.

—Dame Cicely Saunders

In 1948, Cicely Saunders met a man who would change her life. She was a thirty-year-old nurse and social worker, volunteering part time at St. Luke's Hospital in London, an institution that had been founded a half century earlier as a home for the "dying poor." She became captivated by a patient named David Tasma, a Polish Jewish refugee who had escaped from the Warsaw ghetto, worked as a waiter in London, and was now dying of cancer. Through her work and this relationship, she developed an awareness of the suffering and indignity experienced by dying patients and, together with David, shared ideas as to how this could be different. When he died, David bequeathed her £500 (about $23,600 today) to be "a window in your home." It was the beginning of an entirely new type of medical care, a care specifically focused on the needs of the dying. She called it hospice.

The word "hospice" was not new, but this meaning was. The term is derived from the same Latin root as our words "hospital," "hostel," and "hospitality." This Latin term first meant "stranger," but over time usage changed and it came to refer to a host, one who welcomes the stranger. During the medieval era, hospices were inns, boarding houses along pilgrim routes that served as places of rest and refreshment. On these long treks through Europe, many pilgrims became ill, often fatally. The hospices served then as places of care, possible recovery, and often death. The word had been used since the mid-nineteenth century in Britain and Ireland for homes for the dying, places where the poor with nowhere else to go died. What Dr. Saunders did was to create a new connotation of the word "hospice," keeping the welcoming but transforming it from a place to a model, a system of caring for the dying.

Cicely Saunders did not start out in health care. Her initial training was in politics, philosophy, and economics. In 1940, she entered nursing school, but because a back injury prevented her from doing the heavy work that nursing required, she went back to school and qualified as a medical social worker. The years she spent at St. Luke's as part of a staff that cared deeply about the plight of those who were dying in their care demonstrated to her the impotence of the care system in the face of the patients' ongoing pain. Knowing that the medical establishment would be resistant to hearing the ideas of an upstart social worker, she went to medical school. She then practiced for seven years at St. Joseph's hospice in east London, listening to patients, keeping meticulous records, and monitoring the results of her treatments to relieve pain and other symptoms.[1]

One of the first practices she challenged was the method of prescribing opioids, strong pain relievers like morphine. The prevailing practice had been to only use these drugs, given as injection, when the pain appeared severe, when it seemed to the doctor or nurse that the patient was hurting enough to "deserve" relief. The common result was that patients were either in unrelieved pain or briefly asleep after a drug dose. Then, as now, what most people "knew" about opioids was that they were addictive and dangerous. What Dr. Saunders recognized was that patients were the only ones who knew how bad their pain was and that their reports could be trusted. Since an oral dose of morphine lasts about four hours, she decided to give doses that often, by the clock, not by waiting until the pain had recurred. She also added smaller doses of analgesics between the scheduled doses if the pain "broke through." This simple yet revolutionary idea, when put into practice, demonstrated that pain could be effectively relieved, and when this was accomplished, the patients could function more fully, engage with others more effectively, and contend with their other symptoms as well as the hopes and fears that came from the fact that they were terminally ill. In other words, they were able to live.

In 1967, Dr. Saunders opened St. Christopher's Hospice in London, incorporating what she had learned into its structure and operations. The architecture included a sheet of glass at the entrance honoring Mr. Tasma's bequest. She saw the mission of St. Christopher's as providing not only excellent patient care but also a center of education and research, focusing on improving symptom relief and broadening the appreciation of this knowledge into the larger world of health care.

Dr. Saunders identified that pain was not just a physical phenomenon. Morphine was not all that was needed. She described "total pain," the hurting that occurred in the physical body, the emotional psyche, the spiritual depths, and the surrounding family. She attacked it with a model of care aimed at all facets of life that contributed to that pain. Effective analgesia was, of course, a priority. But she recognized that it takes a team of skilled and caring professionals to do the job completely: bedside nursing to promote symptom relief and bodily integrity; social work to address financial and family concerns and to mobilize community resources; and clergy to provide empathic listening, words of comfort and advice, and insight into the realms of meaning and transcendence. She extended this care model into the community, providing services for patients dying in their homes, and she introduced family support during the patient's illness and also after the death. Her ideas remain the bedrock of modern hospice care as well as its sister discipline, palliative care. In 1979, Queen Elizabeth II named Dr. Saunders a Dame Commander of the Order of the British Empire.

Dr. Saunders's model of care spread across the Atlantic, finding fertile ground especially among nurses who were frustrated by the way the medical establishment seemed to be both overtreating and abandoning the dying. Florence Wald, dean of the School of Nursing at Yale University, served as the catalyst and, with a small group of colleagues, founded Connecticut Hospice in 1974, modeling their program after St. Christopher's but adapting it to the local medical and social culture. This was two decades before the SUPPORT study (see chapter 1) would formally describe the suffering and intensive care endured by dying patients, but these visionaries and many like them recognized that a more humane way of dying was possible. Hospices began springing up around the country—small, mostly volunteer agencies, often associated with hospitals or religious institutions. As most of these relied mainly on donations and volunteers, the services offered varied widely.

A watershed moment in the care of the dying in the United States came in 1982 when the US Congress and President Reagan enacted the Medicare Hospice Benefit (MHB). This established a funding mechanism for hospice care and set standards for the organizational structures and for patient care. The MHB, as initially conceived, envisioned a "typical" hospice patient as someone with advanced cancer and no further treatment options, one whose course after hospice enrollment would be manageable, predictable, and short. In the ensuing decades, medical (e.g., AIDS epidemic, hospice for multiple other illnesses), financial (e.g., drug costs, federal budget deficits), and demographic (e.g., aging baby boomers) pressures have resulted in tweaks and modifications of the regulations, but the MHB continues to define how hospice care is provided in the United States.

THE BENEFITS OF THE MEDICARE HOSPICE BENEFIT

For a hospice agency to receive Medicare payment for their services, they need to adhere to federal standards, which are termed "conditions of participation."[2] Insurance companies, Medicaid programs, and managed care organizations all developed methods to pay for hospice care, generally basing their benefits on the federal program. Initially a simple set of guidelines, the "COPs" and their associated regulations have evolved into a cumbersome and dizzying set of rules, requiring hospice agencies to increasingly shift scarce resources to ensure compliance.

There are only two criteria for someone to qualify for and receive the Medicare Hospice Benefit. First, they must have a terminal prognosis—that is, two separate physicians must certify that they will most likely die within the next six months. The second criterion is that they must accept the MHB as the coverage for the medical conditions contributing to that terminal prognosis. In practical terms, this generally means that they abandon medical treatments aimed at disease control—treatments like chemotherapy, dialysis, or hospitalization for exacerbations of heart failure or chronic lung disease. Instead, their treatment focuses on the alleviation of symptoms and suffering as well as anticipation of and preparation for the end of their lives. This "one or the other but not both" approach has delayed acceptance of hospice care by many patients as well as their physicians, but virtually every hospice professional avers that the most common comment from patients and families after experience with hospice is "we should have done this much sooner."

Before outlining the details of what hospice care is like, let me take on one huge and prevalent misconception about hospice care, that it involves "giving up" on treatment and "letting nature take its course." Most people assume that moving to hospice care means that death will come sooner than if they kept "fighting," but this is not true. In the best studies that have been done, patients who enter hospice care do not die sooner than those who do not. And in addition to life not being shortened, it is usually better. The energy that had previously been expended in fighting disease and putting up with adverse effects of medical treatment can now be channeled into experiencing and living the remaining days or months focused on the people, places, and ideas that are most important. Living better while living just as long is sometimes called the "hospice magic."

So how does this magic happen? Hospice care is provided by a team of professionals who, with the patient and family, identify symptoms, problems, and priorities and develop a plan for addressing them. Note that the unit of hospice care is the patient and their family, with family being whoever that is as identified by the patient. The MHB is designed assuming that the preponderance of the day-to-day, hour-by-hour care will be provided by that family. Each hospice agency certified by Medicare must at a minimum provide the services of a team of professionals: physician, nurse, social worker, spiritual care coordinator, nursing assistant, and bereavement counselor as well as speech, physical, and occupational therapists for patients whose symptoms require them. In addition, hospice agencies must recruit, train, and deploy a cadre of volunteers whose responsibilities may range from stuffing envelopes to providing hours of bedside presence, allowing a family caregiver to shop for groceries, run errands, or attend church. Trained volunteers may also keep vigil with a family witnessing the very end of the life of their loved one. While the listed required services are paid for by Medicare, hospice teams may also include art, music, or massage therapists as well as practitioners of energy therapies, mindfulness techniques, or other complementary approaches, with or without cost to the patient.

One of Dr. Saunders's valuable contributions was her recognition that, while her patients may have had cancer, heart failure, or tuberculosis, their underlying lethal disease was not the most important problem. The primary diagnosis, the imperative that drove the care of all her patients, was that they were dying. The medical care of the dying patient requires a set of skills derived from multiple other specialties. Hospice physicians have chosen to acquire expertise in the management of pain and other symptoms, and an increasing number have obtained board certification. The job of the hospice medical director (HMD) is to oversee the care of the patients, to ensure its quality, and to establish that each patient meets the criteria for hospice—that is, that they are more likely than not to die within the next six months.

Hospice patients choose who their own doctor will be; many wish for their primary care physician, or a specialist such as their oncologist, to continue the responsibility for their care, but often they choose to have the HMD or another physician employed by the hospice agency to follow them. A physician with whom one has a long-standing relationship may possess in-depth understanding of the patient's needs, support system, and values. But, as discussed in chapter 1, some doctors do not possess the interest or expertise to manage their patients well at the end of their lives, so, in these cases, it is in the patient's best interest to transfer their care to a hospice physician. Sometimes a patient's own doctor will want to remain in charge of the overall care but ask the hospice physician to manage pain and other physical symptoms. The staff of a hospice agency might have preferences as to the physicians they work with, but they should be flexible to accommodate patient wishes. The patient carries the authority to have the physician of their choice care for them, if that doctor is willing to do so.

The hospice nurse acts as an educator and case manager. Nurses review the medication regimen and instruct the patient and family about the pills they are taking, what they are, how they should be taken, what they are supposed to do, and what side effects to watch for. They make frequent visits, answer questions as they arise, and assess how the patient's symptoms are being managed and how well the family is coping and keeping up with the demands of care. The nurse acts as liaison and advocate in the relationship between the patient and the physician. We saw in chapter 2 that the nurse is seen by the patient and family as the medical expert who also provides the time and skill to listen and respond to their needs and concerns. Many hospice nurses have obtained additional training and certification in the field of hospice and palliative nursing. A good hospice nurse is the linchpin of excellent end-of-life care.

Hospice nursing assistants provide hands-on personal care and instruct the family and patient in how to do this themselves as well as on the techniques of skin care, safe mobilization, and other issues of day-to-day living. As nursing assistants see patients more often than other members of the team, and often when the patient is at their most vulnerable, they are likely to be the ones who identify impending problems or issues that have been overlooked by others. I have been impressed by how often those working as nursing assistants, a position society views as a demeaning or entry-level job with a low pay scale, see their work as a calling and demonstrate their dedication to it by honing their skills and taking certification exams. I have heard from several nursing assistant colleagues that they particularly value the time spent bathing patients, as it is often during those unprotected and private times that patients open up in ways they don't feel comfortable with in front of family or other caregivers.

Social workers provide indispensable attention, advocacy, and advice on practical matters like advance directives, finances, and funeral planning. They may also be helpful in identifying other sources of assistance or support for the patient and family during this time. Many social workers are excellent resources for sorting through and resolving family conflicts.

Much of the "total pain" that Dr. Saunders identified lies in the realms of faith and meaning. Spiritual care professionals, sometimes called chaplains, who are trained in and attuned to this kind of pain can provide a safe outlet for the patient's deep questions and assist them in finding purpose and healing, within themselves, with other persons, and with the transcendent. We will explore questions of religion and spirituality at the end of life further in chapter 6.

Bereavement counselors are invaluable to surviving loved ones struggling with their grief and learning to live without the departed one. Bereavement services are provided to the surviving family for at least thirteen months after the death of the patient and can take the form of individual or group sessions or art, music, or craft-based expression. Like all the hospice staff we have described here, their services are part of the MHB. All are essential to produce the hospice magic.

As was mentioned above, hospice care is most often delivered in the home setting, where most Americans desire to live the end of their lives. While not every family can mobilize the physical and emotional resources to provide care to a dying relative, those who do often find that this becomes a gift they can give to one they care about, a method of expressing love, and an experience of profound meaning.

About one-third of Americans die in extended care facilities, and they also can benefit from hospice care. In this situation, the facility staff augment or even assume the functions of the "family" for the patient as well as being the providers of day-to-day care. In addition, many hospice agencies have an inpatient hospice unit. While these may provide residential care for a few patients with no other option, their major focus is on "intensive hospice care," management of symptoms or other crises that cannot be controlled in the home setting. Wherever the patient is located, one goal is to make that location feel like "home."

Hospice care, under the Medicare benefit, is funded by a per diem payment to the hospice agency, intended to cover all care related to the terminal prognosis. All the professional staff listed above are paid out of these funds. In addition, the hospice provides patients with whatever durable medical equipment (hospital bed, commode, wheelchair, oxygen, etc.) is needed and appropriate. Another significant benefit is that all medications that are related to the terminal state are provided. Hospice agencies may charge a nominal co-pay for these drugs, but most do not. This drug coverage is of particular value to those without other prescription coverage and avoids the "doughnut holes" of many Medicare Part D plans.

Many myths have grown up about hospice care. One that I commonly hear from other physicians is "the only thing hospice does is give my patients morphine." Patients referred to hospice often have a high burden of symptoms that need to be addressed quickly; they may be suffering on multiple levels. If the pain, shortness of breath, and other physical symptoms are not relieved quickly, addressing those other areas of the patient's total pain will be impossible. Hospice physicians are experts in symptom management and are more comfortable in using powerful medicines at higher doses than many other clinicians. They are also experts in knowing how to balance the effects of these medicines with the patient's needs, goals, and safety. The opioid epidemic rampant in many parts of the United States has made these skills even more important.

Perhaps the most prevalent societal myth about hospice is that it is about dying. When patients express that they are "not ready" for hospice, what they are often really saying is that they are not ready to die. We have already noted that hospice care does not shorten life. The public perception persists, though, that one goes to hospice to die and even possibly to have one's death hastened. It is not uncommon for a patient, once their pain and suffering are being better managed, to say, "Okay, I'm ready for the pill." The "pill" is presumably the euthanasia drug that they expect the hospice to provide when they request it. Of course, there is no such pill. We will discuss medical aid in dying in the next chapter, but the prevalent hospice position is to neither hasten nor delay dying. As was emphasized above, the goal of hospice to provide a good death is achieved by maximizing the quality of the time available— that is, hospice is not about death but about life.

What Is It Like to Go on Hospice?

For the patient choosing hospice care, the initial few days can be hectic. A representative from the agency, often a nurse, will meet with the patient and family to describe how hospice care is provided, answer questions, review the necessary forms, and often assist in obtaining a portable DNR form or other advance directives. Note that most hospices do not require a DNR order, but for most patients this is consistent with their goals. A patient has a choice of which hospice agency to sign up with, and some choose to meet with representatives from two or three agencies before enrolling with one provider. We will discuss how to select a hospice agency at the end of this chapter.

Several questions will be asked of the patient and family. One, as mentioned above, is who the attending physician will be. If the patient is hospitalized at the time of referral, the doctor of record will probably be a hospitalist, who will sign the certification forms and prescribe the medications but will not continue to care for the patient after discharge. Another question that sometimes takes people by surprise is who they have chosen as a funeral director and if they have made arrangements. It is not necessary to have those arrangements made to be admitted to hospice, but patients and families are usually encouraged to at least make a choice of provider before the moment of death.

The next needs to be addressed are the delivery of medications and equipment. If the patient is to be cared for at home, there may be furniture to be moved and other rearrangements to be made to create a space for a hospital bed and whatever other supplies will be needed. Sometimes this space is in the patient's own bedroom, but often the choice is to establish the "sick room" in a more central living area so that the patient can continue to be an active part of the family's life. Several people will visit in the first couple of days; Medicare requires an evaluation by each of the professional disciplines very soon after hospice admission. The hospice nurse will usually spend a few hours evaluating the patient's symptoms and needs, setting up medicines and schedules for nursing assistants and other care professionals, and teaching the family how to perform all the new tasks that will be required of them and how to contact the hospice in an emergency. The social worker will review patient and family safety, help set up care schedules, sort through financial needs, coordinate with any other agencies involved, and review and assist in executing any needed advance directives. The spiritual care coordinator will inquire about the patient's religious affiliation or preference and any other spiritual or existential questions. The patient and family are also asked how they want this kind of support to be provided: through the patient or family's faith community, the hospice chaplain, both, or, if the patient requests, not at all. Sometimes the agency staff will try to combine these visits to most efficiently address all the needs and also limit the amount of time the family must spend in these meetings. The last period of life is often a dynamic time, with fluctuating and sometimes sudden symptoms and needs, so hospice care must be a flexible, ongoing process, with all disciplines involved for the entire course. These first visits, with the establishment of a coherent and comprehensive plan of care, are essential to be able to respond to crises when they arise.

Trivia That Is Sometimes Important

There are many "nuts and bolts" of hospice care, the arcana of the MHB, that occasionally impact the care of an individual patient. The first regards medications; hospice agencies are required to provide all medications for the "palliation and management of the terminal illness and related conditions as identified in the hospice plan of care." Hospice agencies vary in how they interpret this regulation, especially as far as what constitutes a "related condition." The hospice medical director establishes what medical conditions are present that contribute to a patient's terminal prognosis and then which of the patient's medicines will be covered by hospice; the remainder are the responsibility of the patient, though these will usually be covered by an existing Medicare Part D plan or other prescription coverage. For example, for a patient dying of lung cancer, the hospice agency would pay for the pain medicines, laxatives, oxygen, and nebulized breathing treatments but not for any drugs taken for ongoing high blood pressure. Most hospices employ a formulary or preferred drug list, like those any other pharmacy benefit provider maintains. If a drug is needed and is safe and effective, it must be provided. But if there is a less expensive alternative just as safe and effective, the hospice has the right to cover the less expensive one but not the other. From pharmaceutical and medical standpoints, this is appropriate and effective care. Sometimes, for whatever reason, a patient prefers to stay on the pill they've used before, and they have the right to do so even if the hospice will not cover it. If that patient is on Medicare, though, by electing the MHB, they have given up other coverage for the terminal conditions. This means that if they want to continue a noncovered drug, this is the exception in that their Part D plan will also probably not cover it. It is quite rare for this to develop into an issue of conflict, especially if the hospice benefit is explained and understood; the goal is the right drug for the right patient at the right time.

The MHB is a capitated health plan—that is, the hospice agency receives a specified amount of money for each patient-day, no matter what it costs them to provide care for the patient. Because of this, hospices sometimes must make tough decisions about expensive treatments. One common example of this is blood transfusions. Patients with leukemias, lymphomas, and similar cancers often receive blood transfusions because the body's ability to make new blood is impaired by the disease and treatment. During disease-directed therapy, transfusions of red blood cells are necessary to keep the patient functioning and to lessen symptoms of anemia, such as fatigue and shortness of breath. When these patients enter hospice care, these symptoms may persist and be alleviated by further transfusions. Therefore, transfusion is a symptom-relieving measure that is clearly related to the conditions causing the terminal prognosis and therefore is the responsibility of the hospice. But the transfusion need for a patient like this can, combined with the other services the hospice must provide, cost far more than the agency receives. Hospice organizations deal with this in one of several ways. Some hospices have a policy against giving transfusions and do not admit patients who wish to continue them. This can be appropriate, as a hospice should only admit a patient if they have adequate resources to care for them. Some programs provide transfusion but only in their own inpatient unit, thus eliminating the expense of sending the patient to a hospital. Some will cover transfusion on a "time-limited trial" basis—that is, periodically evaluating, maybe after each transfusion procedure, whether receiving blood is still producing symptom relief. Hospices that do provide transfusion use the patient's symptoms, rather than a lab test value, as the reason for giving blood and will continue it only if the transfusions continue to make a real difference in the patient's symptoms and quality of life.

The MHB provides for four levels of daily hospice care, with a different reimbursement level for each. The most common is routine daily care, the ongoing care provided in the patient's residence. The second is respite care, up to five consecutive days, for the needs of the family caregivers. This usually involves a home care patient being relocated to a hospice facility or nursing home for the few days of the respite. The third level, continuous care, is provided when an uncontrolled symptom or other crisis erupts that requires frequent professional evaluation and intervention; during continuous care the agency places staff, usually a nurse, in the home for at least eight hours daily. The most intensive level is general inpatient care (GIP), for a patient with symptoms that cannot be managed at the patient's residence. Many hospices have their own inpatient facilities for this purpose, but others contract with hospitals or skilled nursing facilities to provide this care. Continuous and GIP care are both intended to be used for no more than several days.

The final and perhaps most confusing regulatory piece is the certification process. The COP requires that the hospice agency, specifically the medical director, certify that an enrolled patient meets the criterion of being terminally ill—that is, that if the condition progresses at the expected rate, survival will likely be less than six months. This certification must be repeated at specified intervals, termed "benefit periods." The first and second benefit periods are ninety days each; these are followed by an unlimited number of sixty-day benefit periods. Before the start of each new benefit period, the medical director must again certify terminal prognosis and compose a narrative statement arguing why that is the case. For the third and each subsequent benefit period, this narrative statement must be preceded by a face-to-face visit by a physician or nurse practitioner employed by the hospice agency to provide firsthand evidence supporting the prognosis. If it is determined, as in the case of Dorothy in the previous chapter, that the terminal prognosis no longer exists, the patient must be discharged from hospice care. When I made face-to-face visits, the patient or a family member would often quip, "Well, I guess the government doesn't think I'm dying fast enough!" But the goal of recertification is not to save Medicare money or, on the other hand, to keep the hospice census high, but to be sure that the patient is receiving the level of care most appropriate for their situation.

SIMON

I wondered if Simon owned a mirror. Did he know what he looked like? The cancer had probably destroyed his sense of smell so that he didn't notice the stench that permeated the house, that I could still taste an hour after I left him. The cancer had started in the right maxillary sinus, the part of the skull just below the right eye. By the time I met him, after he had been referred to hospice care, the malignancy and effects of treatment had eaten away a three-inch hole through the skin and bones of the face and had destroyed the eye socket and palate on the right side of his mouth. He could still speak and swallow, but when he drank, some of the liquid flowed sideways out of the hole, where it mixed with the liquefying dead tissue lining the cavity and dripped onto the floor. Simon managed the efflux by carpeting the area under his chair with newspaper.

His appearance was repellent, but Simon was much more than his disease; in fact, though the cancer was flagrantly conspicuous, it had little to do with his personhood. He was a military veteran and proud of the fact. He had worked as a letter carrier and, though he was not religious, he talked about his job being like that of a priest. He took time to get to know people on his route, to talk with them and learn their stories, including the dark sides of what was happening in their lives, as he placed their letters, wafer-like, into their hands or mail slots.

Simon had little physical pain. The process that destroyed his face also destroyed the nerves as it went. There were now tumors in his lungs as the cancer sought out other fertile ground from which to continue the gradual destruction of his body. But he had living to do. He went, Phantom-of-the-Opera-like, to Walmart when he needed groceries or supplies. He wouldn't let us come on Sunday because that's when Antoinette came to visit—Antoinette who, maybe among other things, cooked for him "between the sheets."

HOW TO CHOOSE A HOSPICE AGENCY

Though the MHB conditions of participation establish nationwide rules and standards for hospice agencies, there is considerable variation in the way those regulations are interpreted by hospice providers. As a colleague puts it, "If you've seen one hospice program, you've seen one hospice program." In the early days of hospice in the United States, agencies usually served populations based on demographics, city or county of residence, hospital service area, or even religion or ethnicity. But now, especially in more populated areas, multiple hospice organizations offer service in competition with each other. A small faith-based organization will not have the same culture or provide service in the same way as a large national for-profit hospice chain, but both can provide excellent hospice services to the majority of dying patients. A good deal of the time, a hospice referral is made to an agency most commonly used by the referring physician, social worker, or facility, and usually that is just fine. Sometimes, though, there are good reasons to choose one agency over another.

The first consideration is recommendations and reputation. Is there an agency that has been used with positive results by a friend or other family member? Is there a hospice organization that carries a good reputation in your area? What provider was recommended by your doctor, hospital, or nursing home social worker? Physicians and facilities often have preferences based on experience. Note, though, that what doctors like, such as ease of the referral process, effective communication, and few emergency calls, may not be what is most important to you. And some health care institutions choose "preferred" providers for reasons most advantageous to the facility, not necessarily the patients. That being said, if your doctor tells you "this is who I would choose for my own care if I needed it," that is a strong endorsement. Also, if your hospice coverage is through a private insurance firm, there may be significant financial repercussions if you choose a provider not in their approved network.

Second, how can you assess the quality of the agency and the staff? Is the agency certified by Medicare? (If not, they can't get paid by Medicare, so most are.) Have they obtained certification by The Joint Commission? Joint Commission certification is a voluntary process, like the one used in hospitals, that establishes how well the hospice agency complies with standards of effective and safe patient care. Many hospices use the Family Evaluation of Hospice Care (FEHC), or a similar tool, as a self-evaluation mechanism. The FEHC survey is sent to the bereaved family several weeks after the patient's death, querying numerous aspects of the care provided. Agencies are compared with regional and national norms. While FEHC scores are not intended to be used as a publicly reported measure of quality, participation in the process is evidence of an agency emphasis on quality. In 2014, the Center for Medicare and Medicaid Services began collecting specific measures of quality care from hospices and began reporting these measures publicly in 2017 on the "hospice compare" web page.[3]

What about the medical director and hospice physicians? The traditional mechanism or assurance of physician competence in a medical specialty is board certification. While board certification is not essential for a doctor to practice quality hospice medicine, it does demonstrate a commitment to excellence. Whether a hospice agency expects their physicians to be certified and how many of their doctors have achieved and maintained certification could reflect its vision of superior care. In particular, the medical director (sometimes called chief medical officer or a similar title) should have the personal commitment to superior practice that certification illustrates. A related question is whether agency doctors are members of the American Academy of Hospice and Palliative Medicine, the professional scientific organization of the field.

Does the agency encourage staff to demonstrate excellence by pursuing professional certification? How many of the hospice nurses have obtained Certified Hospice and Palliative Nurse (CHPN) status? Similarly, how many nursing assistants (CHN), social workers (CHP-SW), and chaplains (BCC-HPCC) are certified?

How long has the agency been providing hospice care? What is its service area? Is it associated with a hospital or health system that you have used for your medical care? Does it have its own inpatient unit, and, if so, is it located close to where you live? Is it a nonprofit entity or part of a for-profit corporation? Corporate culture can foster efficiency and innovation and provide a consistent product, but some have raised concerns as to whose interests are paramount, the patient's or the stockholders', though evidence that profit-making status affects care quality is conflicting. On the other hand, nonprofit agencies rely on donations to supplement Medicare and insurance payments to support their mission. How often, for example, do families request memorial gifts be given to the hospice agency or that they become donors themselves?

Is there specific religious or philosophical emphasis in the agency's mission? Many hospices were started with the admirable purpose of meeting the needs of the suffering, and these religious underpinnings provide a richness of culture and sense of servanthood. But occasionally this can bring along doctrinal baggage, such as opposition to stopping "ordinary" measures such as tube feeding or prohibiting aggressive comfort procedures such as palliative sedation (discussed in the next chapter). Also, in states that have legalized physician medical aid in dying, hospices vary as to their acceptance of or involvement in this practice.

Size matters sometimes. As discussed above, more expensive drugs and treatments, even if aimed squarely at patient comfort, can create financial challenges for hospice organizations. Agencies with a larger patient census may be able to have a more individualized approach to these care decisions.

How do procedures play out in real life? For example, hospices are required to provide care around the clock, but practices vary. If a family member calls in the middle of the night, will they speak with a nurse or with a remote answering service? Is the agency's on-call system effective in controlling new symptoms and solving problems or is it more often used to put off intervention until the next morning? Deaths, like births, seem to avoid normal business hours; how does the hospice allow for this?

No hospice agency is perfect, and none meets every need, but good hospice care is widely available. For patients and families, the face of the organization is the staff that they meet. For most patients in most situations, a competent and caring hospice nurse, a gentle and efficient nursing assistant, and respectful and compassionate counselors are more important than corporate structure or administrative policies. As an example of this, the nonprofit hospice agency that very recently provided care for my mother-in-law lists ten physicians on their website, only two of whom are certified in HPM. The agency uses the FEHC process to evaluate its quality but is not certified by The Joint Commission. Some of their procedures were not exactly what I, as a hospice professional, would have preferred. But the services that my wife's mother received were excellent, personal, professional, and caring. I would highly recommend them to anyone living in their service area. And, yes, her family did request memorial contributions go to them.

✳ ✳ ✳

Simon kept on living, and so did the cancer. The chasm grew, and the entire right side of his upper jaw, nose, and skull gradually disappeared onto the soggy, befouled newspaper. In the depths of the wound, the gray coverings of his brain were clearly visible. By now the reek was detectable half a block away. When his hospice nurse called his oncologist for new orders, the reply was "Is he still alive?" Simon amazed us all; his body continued to survive despite unthinkable damage, and his personhood continued to challenge and teach us about living with equanimity and even grace.

There is no other care model except hospice that could have allowed Simon to stay in his home and live his life as he chose. I was amazed that, despite an extended course with a horrific disease, Simon never seemed to exhibit signs of suffering. He was somehow able to divorce himself from or maybe rise above what for many would be intolerable. And each of us who were involved in his care, who risked the stench and the ugliness, encountered wholeness and even beauty.

PALLIATIVE CARE

The discoveries that Dame Cicely Saunders made in the care of the dying are effective for any person with significant symptoms and suffering related to injury or illness, no matter what their survival prognosis. Unfortunately, in the United States, the MHB established a payment mechanism for this team-based expert care only for those with a terminal prognosis. The application of the ideas born in hospice to patients who are not at the end of their lives is called palliative care. Palliative care can and should be delivered alongside of or incorporated with disease-directed therapy. The goals of palliative care are relieving pain and other physical symptoms, establishing goals of care, communicating those goals and priorities, and empowering individuals with serious illness to live well and even thrive. The SUPPORT study and patient reports alluded to earlier in chapter 1 accentuate the need for this approach in the American medical system.

Hospital-based palliative care was pioneered in North America by Dr. Balfour Mount at the Royal Victoria Hospital in Montreal in the 1970s. Dr. Mount used the culture and resources of an academic teaching hospital to establish palliative care as a scientific discipline. Throughout the United States, palliative care teams have been developed in hospitals as well as in numerous outpatient venues. Good palliative care, like hospice, requires a team approach, but to this point there is no established funding mechanism; billings by palliative care physicians or nurse practitioners are not adequate to support the team members' salaries. This means that hospitals and health systems need to make a financial investment. Fortunately, more and more of these as well as some insurance plans are recognizing both the need for and value of palliative care. This has occurred partly because of patient demand. These forward-thinking institutions are finding their investment paying off in terms of improved patient outcomes and more efficient use of other expensive resources, like intensive care units.

Scientific studies demonstrating the value of and best ways of delivering palliative care are ongoing. One early report, though, led to surprising findings. Patients with metastatic non-small-cell lung cancer who were referred to a palliative care team as they were beginning their cancer treatment experienced improved quality of life, fewer depressive symptoms, and less use of aggressive end-of-life care. These findings, while confirming value, were hardly unexpected to the palliative care community. The surprise, though, was that despite receiving less chemotherapy and other aggressive treatment, the group who received early palliative care lived longer than the other patients![4] Maybe good symptom control helped patients maintain their strength to tolerate chemotherapy better. Maybe the palliative care team provided an additional support system, allowing patients to keep involved with life. More and more cancer centers and oncology practices are including palliative care expertise in the treatment of patients with advanced cancer, and the American Society of Clinical Oncology now recommends palliative care consultation for all patients with advanced cancers.[5]

Palliative care services are expanding and proliferating, but the need still outweighs availability. Palliative care is appropriate and should be available throughout the course of a serious illness. If you or a loved one are being treated for a serious, potentially life-threatening illness like cancer, heart failure, chronic lung disease, or a degenerative neurologic disorder, ask your doctor or hospital about the availability of a palliative care team. It might just change your life.

4

SUFFERING

How long must I continue to suffer such intolerable pain?
When will I be permitted to accept "sweet peace" or even to ask
for it?

—Sigmund Freud

I was having a bit of difficulty keeping my lunch down as we were talking, our conversation occasionally punctuated by his retching. I don't do well with vomiting, so when Bob told me his primary request was that he not "puke to death," I understood him "loud and clear and in living color." Bob had cancer that had started in the lower esophagus, at its connection with the stomach, and he had experienced recurrent vomiting throughout his disease course. Now, with the cancer spread extensively throughout his body, he recognized both that he was dying and that vomiting was part of his life. He did not want it to be part of his death.

Bob owned a small business and was used to having things go his way. He shared his comfortable home with Barbara, his wife, and Captain, their champion Irish setter. Their retreat during the winter was a hilltop villa in Costa Rica. Bob had consulted a Buddhist death coach in an attempt to make sense of and even direct his dying. Bob and Barbara welcomed the hospice team wholeheartedly; we were the experts and had been highly recommended by a family friend. He and I reviewed his symptoms, the treatment he had received, what had been tried for the vomiting, and what effect the different medicines and procedures had produced. Of course, he wanted as much relief as possible now, but he would not allow me to use medicines that would make him sleepy, as it was more important to him to be alert, to be able to interact with his family, to accomplish his end-of-life work. He wanted to know that later, when his work was completed, when his body was finally overmastered by his disease, when all that was left for him to do was to die, that he would be able to accomplish it without the physical misery that had plagued his existence for the past several months. He gave me the assignment to work with him on a plan to manage that time when it came; my commitment to him was that I would do everything within the limits of medicine and law to relieve his suffering and allow his death to be symptom free and, hopefully, peaceful.

He was the one who brought up palliative sedation, a procedure in which the physician prescribes medications to produce a sleep state for a patient with refractory symptoms. He wanted to know the details about how we could do this in his home, what planning would need to be done ahead, and how much time would be needed to get the medicines going after he had decided that it was time for them. I pointed out to him that the midazolam or phenobarbital we would use might not stop him from vomiting. Since he would be asleep, he would not be aware of it, but his family could still see his body retching. I also told him that he probably would not die immediately after the sedating medicines were started but could linger unconscious for some hours to days. Barbara understood her husband's desires and agreed with the plan. And so did I. Bob wanted to die as he had lived, in control as much as possible and able to make that final decision of when it was time so say good-bye, to go to sleep.

WHAT IS SUFFERING?

Patients nearing the end of their lives commonly say that it is not dying that they dread but suffering. Often this imagined horror is unremitting physical pain, and that is undoubtedly dreadful and can produce profound distress. Suffering can arise from physical symptoms like pain, but it encompasses the merely physical experience, expanding into all parts of one's being to produce an overall sense of anguish. Suffering is an essentially human experience that is different from, and much more complex than, a symptom like pain or vomiting. While it is difficult to define suffering, we know it when we experience it. In his landmark book, *The Nature of Suffering and the Goals of Medicine*,[1] Dr. Eric Cassell points out that while an organ or body part—a bone, liver, or heart—can experience pain, only a person can suffer. A person has an identity, a past, a set of values, a group of relationships that all impact how they perceive symptoms and situations. Some people have excruciating pain but seem to live with it, while others with less intense symptoms are overwhelmed by them. Suffering can even occur in the absence of physical pain. Suffering encounters the meaning of what is being experienced, is intimate with fear and dread, and has a forward-looking focus. The suffering person may say, "If this keeps up, I will not be able to endure it." This is a telling statement, as at the moment they say this, they are managing to endure it. It is the fear of being overcome by their distress that produces suffering. Dr. Cassell says that suffering occurs "when an impending destruction of the person is perceived; it continues until the threat of disintegration has passed or until the integrity of the person can be restored."

To illustrate the distinction between pain and suffering, imagine two women, both thirty-two years old, lying in beds in the same hospital. Both have large, tightly swollen abdomens and endure intermittent spasms of wrenching pain, its intensity rated ten out of ten, causing them to scream, "Just make it stop!" One of these women has ovarian cancer that has spread extensively throughout her abdominal cavity, causing an intestinal blockage.

With the movement of each bubble of bowel gas, the pain is excruciating. Each throb reminds her that she has cancer, that there is nothing more that can be done to fix it, and that she will die soon. The other woman is giving birth to her first child. Her pain is just as severe, but each contraction tells her she is just that much closer to holding her infant. These women's physical pains are identical, but the meanings are profoundly different, as are their degrees of suffering.

Put on a Happy Face

We don't like to look at suffering, at least not for very long. We are drawn to new misfortune; rubberneckers slow down to check out the crash in the oncoming lanes, creating traffic jams. But if we have to look at adversity for more than a few seconds, as in a commercial soliciting donations to provide famine relief or to fight animal cruelty, we flip the channel. One measure of dignity in death is how much distress a person exhibits to observers. Patients commonly try to assume a stoic attitude, especially when "important" visitors arrive; they underestimate their symptoms to "please" the doctor; they want to show just how well they are managing their agony.

Nineteenth-century French writer Alphonse Daudet contracted syphilis when he was seventeen and died of it forty years later. As the disease progressed, invading his nervous system, he developed excruciating and unremitting pain. He noted his symptoms and narrated the experiences of fellow patients; these have been assembled in an honest, descriptive, and brief volume titled *In the Land of Pain*.[2] He noted the suffering his pain caused: "Pain finds its way everywhere, into my vision, my feelings, my sense of judgement; it's an infiltration." He observed how others tired of him talking about what he was feeling. He wrote, "Pain is always new to the sufferer, but loses its originality for those around him. Everyone will get used to it except me."[3]

The only one who can assess or measure suffering is the person who is enduring it. And even they may delude themselves, thinking, "Well, maybe I'm making too much of this." After all, big boys and girls don't cry. We've been taught to play hurt, suck it up, walk it off. All we ask of the suffering is that they do it in silence. When a dying patient is told to try to not talk about it or to look on the bright side, it adds yet one more layer to the suffering, that of loneliness.

Hiding the suffering doesn't solve anything; it only makes it worse. Suffering eases only when its sources become less threatening, when meaning is discovered, when integrity is restored. Thankfully, many suffering people, even those facing the end of their lives, can find meaning and recover a degree of wholeness. For some, though, the energy and time this requires are simply unavailable. For them, must the remainder of their existence be one of unremitting distress? What options, then, might they have to find relief from what they find unbearable?

OPTIONS FOR UNBEARABLE SUFFERING

Good hospice and palliative care are very effective in relieving symptoms and lessening suffering. One common reason for a hospice team's failure to relieve symptoms and address suffering is that they are unaware of their existence or severity. Americans are conditioned to put up with adversity, not to ask for help. Difficulty coping is seen as a sign of weakness, admitting need as evidence of some character flaw. Another frequent phenomenon is the patient or family trying to please the doctor or nurse, letting on that their treatments are working rather than risk making them unhappy by reporting the truth about what is happening. There were seemingly innumerable times I heard a spouse ask the patient, "What do you mean, you're doing okay? Why don't you tell him what you complain about every day to me?" The hospice team are strangers at the beginning but can be trusted. They will repeatedly ask about what is troubling you, and they honestly want to know the answers.

Occasionally, despite the best efforts of all members of the team, patients still experience distress they perceive as intolerable. As suffering is an intensely personal experience, it can only be assessed by the one living with it. An expert clinician can discover objective data on the extent of disease and cause of symptoms, but the best evidence of pain and suffering is the patient report. Suffering is complex; what is perceived as a light burden for one person may be intolerable for another or even for the same person at a different time, in a different context. But when suffering is profound and persistent, when it infiltrates every waking moment, the sufferer may feel hopeless, trapped by an egregious enemy. The good news is that there are options available, ways to escape from the unendurable. As I found when working with Bob, it is often true that just knowing there is an "escape plan" can itself relieve suffering. I will review four such plans with sequentially increasing controversy and consequences.

Increased Treatment Intensity

The first option is for the doctor and hospice team to increase the aggressiveness of their involvement. Sometimes, continuous care at the patient's home or temporary admission to a hospice inpatient unit, "hospice intensive care," provides the safest and most effective way to quickly lessen symptom severity. Doses of medications can be increased, new drugs started, and ineffective agents stopped. Family interventions may relieve anxiety about the safety and well-being of loved ones to be left behind. Spiritual exploration may discover sources of meaning to sustain one from minute to minute, day to day. This intensive management, with vigorous attention to physical symptoms and other sources of distress, concurrent with caregiver rest and relief of responsibility, can often "reset" the awareness of suffering to a more bearable level.

Palliative Sedation

The increasing intensity of drug treatment of symptoms described above comes with a cost in the form of adverse effects from medications. One of the common side effects is sleepiness, sedation. For some patients this side effect is agreeable; when they are sleeping they are not aware of their pain, nausea, or shortness of breath. Of course, when they are sleeping they are also not eating or drinking, talking with their friends and family, or interacting with their grandchildren. Finding the point of balance between sedation and symptom relief is the dance between the communicative patient and the adroit clinician. Patients may, for example, request that medications be "lightened up" for the celebration of their wedding anniversary or the return of a child from overseas military service. On the other hand, for someone who has lived with unrelenting symptoms, sedation might be very welcome.

For these individuals, like for Bob, when they have reached their last days of life and all that seems to be left is the suffering, they may dread any conscious experience. If symptoms cannot be controlled using even high doses of medications, an alternative exists to control the symptom by decreasing or eliminating consciousness. This technique is called palliative sedation. The medications that are used here, like midazolam (Versed) and phenobarbital, do not treat pain, nausea, or shortness of breath. In the doses used for palliative sedation, they cause the patient to sleep. Some authorities see this as simply more intensive and appropriate symptom management, but most think that palliative sedation is qualitatively different from the aggressive palliative care described in the previous section. A few critics have pointed out that we cannot really know that unconsciousness eliminates suffering, that it may only erase the memory of it, but patient reports and our universal experience with sleep support the assumption that the appropriately sedated patient is not suffering.

Palliative sedation is sometimes used as a temporary measure, providing a "time-out" from the constant onslaughts and perhaps allowing other medicines or interventions to get started, hoping that on awakening a few days later, symptoms will be lessened and the world will look better, like after a good night's sleep. But more often palliative sedation is a procedure reserved for the last days of life, given with the intention of providing unawareness until death occurs. Note that the intent here is different from that described in the parlance of "putting my dog to sleep"—the goal of palliative sedation is relief of suffering, not hastening of death.

On that point, though, some bioethicists and clinicians argue that palliative sedation is not an ethical act. The sedated patient will not be eating or drinking, so if it continues long enough, they might die from malnutrition or dehydration. This valid concern is rarely of practical consequence, however, as patients at this stage usually have minimal intake, anyway. The larger concern is that palliative sedation is essentially a gradual or controlled overdose of medications, one that theoretically could cause death to occur earlier than it would have otherwise.

Traditionally, the ethical defense of palliative sedation has relied on the philosophic argument of "double effect." This moral principle was first articulated by St. Thomas Aquinas in the thirteenth century and envisions an action that has two foreseeable outcomes: a desired (or good) effect, like relief of suffering, and an undesired (or bad) effect, like the hastened death of the patient. This concept says that for the action to be moral, four key conditions must be met: (1) The action itself must be morally good or neutral (prescribing a medicine is a morally neutral act). (2) The desired effect, not the undesired result, must be intended (the physician's intention must be to relieve symptoms, not to hasten death). (3) The desired effect must not be achieved by way of the undesired effect; in other words, relief of suffering must not come about because the patient dies. (4) There must be proportionality between the desired and undesired effect (relief of suffering must be seen as important enough to risk an earlier death. For someone who believes that life must be preserved at all costs, this condition might not be met).

Applying the principle of double effect to aggressive palliative therapies has provided physicians with a time-honored ethical construct to justify their actions. It has been invoked not only regarding palliative sedation but also the use of high doses of opioids to provide adequate pain relief. From a legal standpoint, the Supreme Court of the United States, using logic similar to Aquinas, ruled that, in cases like this, intention matters. In *Vacco v. Quill* (1997), the court, while finding no "right to die," did support laws that permit appropriately aggressive palliative and symptom care, even if that care risked hastening patient death, as long as the physician's intent was to alleviate pain and suffering.

But, of course, human intention is rarely this pure. As a physician, I had to frequently check myself to be sure that my actions were only driven by the intent to relieve suffering. The patient's intention need not be so pure; a patient may well desire palliative sedation with the hope of hastening death, even if they don't say so. Episodes in which the patient appears adequately sedated and peaceful but the family is distressed because life continues are particularly challenging. Caregivers might whisper, "It's okay, go to the light" in the patient's ear. A family member may report that they know that "she is still in pain" and advocate for increased drug dosage. This has been a repeated test for me, as I desire to relieve suffering wherever I find it, but if I keep turning up drug doses because the family is suffering, I cross an ethical line.

But moral questions about palliative sedation turn out to be much simpler than all this. The best data we have show that if a patient is already in the last days of life, palliative sedation, even to unconsciousness, without food or fluid supplementation, does not hasten death.[4] It is, of course, impossible to be certain what effects will occur with any medical procedure in any individual patient, but in general, death occurs when it will; palliative sedation has little to do with when it happens. Therefore, for someone very near the end of their lives, aggressive symptom control measures up to and including palliative sedation can and, when agreed to by the patient, should be used to treat unbearable suffering.

Hospice and palliative care physicians often say that they provide palliative sedation for relief of uncontrollable symptoms. But in practice they vary as to what symptoms "count" as the cause of suffering beyond that which the patient can bear. Medical societies and ethicists also disagree on this point. All agree that severe physical symptoms, like pain and shortness of breath, justify the use of palliative sedation if other aggressive measures have failed. But what about psychological symptoms, like anxiety, depression, and fear? What about spiritual suffering, like unresolved feelings of guilt or loneliness? What about the person for whom the simple experience of life has no meaning, for whom just awakening to another day is the cause of the distress? Obviously good team-based care includes medical and nonpharmacologic approaches to all these, but for the person with just hours to days to live, there may be neither time nor energy for these approaches to be effective. In my experience, in this very terminal situation, our ability to distinguish among all the intricacies of the causes of distress is exceedingly limited. As discussed above, suffering, even unbearable suffering, may have only limited association with physical symptoms. It is suffering, not symptoms, that is the appropriate target for the procedure of palliative sedation. In my view, for a clinician to aver that a patient must continue to experience suffering that they cannot bear simply because their symptoms don't "qualify" for sedation is the exemplar of arrogance and cruelty. The number of families who had watched their loved one thrash about, heard them scream, and who, after initiation of palliative sedation, were now able to spend the last remaining hours with them talking about memories, cherishing peaceful time together, all told me that I am correct.

Voluntarily Shortening Life

While aggressive symptom control is appropriate throughout the course of an illness, palliative sedation, as we have seen, is indicated only in the last days of life. Some terminally ill patients with weeks or months to live still find their suffering intolerable and desire another choice. For them, another option is acceleration of the dying process. Frequently patients decide to stop potentially life-saving therapies. This is a common occurrence for patients entering hospice care, as the goals of care shift from fighting disease and prolonging existence to comfort and quality of life. The decision to stop hemodialysis, chemotherapy, breathing machines, or tube feedings is made knowing that death is likely to be hastened, gradually or abruptly. Patients may also decide to stop medicines they see as keeping them alive, including those designed to prevent major medical events, like blood thinners, cardiac drugs, even insulin. Weighing the benefits and burdens of all drugs is an essential part of end-of-life care, a universal activity for hospice teams, commonly stopping "preventative" and "nonessential" medications for a dying patient. But trying to die sooner by stopping medicines may have unwanted consequences; sometimes what occurs is not hastened death but worsened physical symptoms. Another method to stop life-prolonging therapies is to decide to not start treatment for an intercurrent illness, for example, forgoing antibiotics if an infection occurs.

Suffering patients often consider actively ending their own lives. Virtually everywhere in the United States, suicide is not illegal. One nurse I worked with talked about "garage diagnoses," those illnesses that she claimed would cause her to take her own life with carbon monoxide using engine exhaust fumes. But acts like this, or the use of firearms, overdose, drowning, and so on, are all tragic acts, particularly as they are usually done alone. This is antithetical to the "good death," the dignified passing that most people say they want.

Researchers in New Zealand identified and examined every case of suicide that occurred in persons over sixty-five in that country between mid-2007 and the end of 2012.[5] Of the 214 cases found, 23 had terminal cancer. In extensive review of the records, they found that those who were terminally ill had a much lower prevalence of depression or any contact with mental health services than those without such a disease. Of the 23 terminally ill individuals who committed suicide, the researchers were able to identify an understandable and rational motivation that suggested that the suicidal act was taken for relief of unbearable suffering.

In the United States, suicide is not a criminal act, but when it occurs or is even attempted by members of the general population, it is seen as evidence of mental illness and is considered a tragedy. Patients treated in emergency rooms for intentional drug overdoses, for example, once medically stabilized, are routinely referred for psychiatric evaluation and may even be hospitalized against their will if they are felt to be a "danger to themselves or others." But when the one acting to end their life is already terminally ill, societal and medical opinion is more complex and even conflicted. If a hospice patient exhibits suicidal thinking or actions as evidence of depression or other mental illness, this is a symptom that needs to be alleviated. But when a patient wishes life to end because of their ongoing suffering, this attitude is evidence of realistic, even hopeful thinking. Distinguishing between these is difficult, particularly as they may coexist. Ongoing suffering, severe and persistent enough to cause a patient to desire death, is a tragedy. And, given time and resources, most such suffering can be ameliorated, but time is exactly what the terminally ill patient does not have. So, they may see hastened death as their only viable option.

One approach that the hospice community often talks about is voluntarily stopping eating and drinking (VSED). It is unknown how many people resort to VSED. A study of hospice nurses showed that about a third of them could think of a patient who had done this over the past four years, indicating that this is an unusual but not unheard-of practice.[6] People with terminal illnesses often have accompanying anorexia or loss of appetite and frequently develop cachexia, or loss of body weight, so the thought has been that VSED might be an effortless way to end life.

Given the fact that so many Americans want to control the end of their lives, the rarity of VSED suggests that might not be as easy as it appears. Let's be honest—we like to eat, and most Americans are not familiar or comfortable with the sensation of persistent hunger. Mealtimes with others commonly have emotional and social context and meaning. The experiences of these patients who do intentionally stop food and fluids, as well as of those who for other reasons go on hunger strikes, show that the sensation of hunger abates after a few days but that if no fluid is taken in, thirst persists. Thirst can be helped by keeping the mouth moist, but it is still uncomfortable. Another practical problem is that death may not occur as fast as might be thought or hoped. In the study mentioned above, the patients who chose VSED were already on hospice and had a very short life expectancy. The average survival from the last intake of food and fluids was ten days, and 85 percent had died within fifteen days. For someone with a somewhat longer life expectancy, especially if they take in some fluids with medications or personal hygiene, death would take significantly longer. For terminally ill people with ongoing distress, fearing that it will be never-ending, VSED can be physically and emotionally draining and may increase symptoms before death occurs.

Medical Aid in Dying

On New Year's Day 2014, Brittany Maynard, a twenty-nine-year-old schoolteacher, recently married and planning a family, found out that the cause of her persistent headaches was a brain tumor. Surgery removed most of the tumor, a grade 2 astrocytoma. This is a relatively slow-growing cancer, but even in a healthy young woman lucky enough to have had successful surgery to remove it, the average survival is less than ten years. This kind of news must have been devastating to someone who thought she had a full life ahead of her. But even that wasn't the worst of what was to happen.

Just a few months after surgery, her tumor recurred with a much more malignant character. It was now classified as grade 4, a cancer also known by the more ominous-sounding name I learned in medical school, glioblastoma multiforme. Usual treatment for this cancer would be repeat surgery to remove as much of the tumor as possible, followed by radiation and chemotherapy. Typical complications of treatment include fatigue, hair loss, and impairment of some brain functions. Even with this aggressive treatment regimen, though, prognosis is dismal; most patients die within months. As the cancer progresses, as it always does, it engenders further devastating neurologic symptoms: weakness or paralysis; seizures; loss of ability to speak, swallow, or see; and eventually coma can and frequently do occur. Because of this tragic outlook with even the best standard therapy, most authorities recommend that patients participate in a clinical trial to help evaluate possible new treatments.

Brittany heard this information and considered her options about how to manage her frightening diagnosis and perilous future. She decided against any further medical treatment. She put it this way: "There is no treatment that would save my life, and the recommended treatments would have destroyed the time I had left."[7] Fearing the likelihood of physical and mental impairment and suffering, she and her family moved their residence from California to Oregon, where medical aid in dying or, as she termed it, "death with dignity," was legal. She wrote, "I do not want to die. But I am dying. And I want to die on my own terms." On November 1, 2014, in her Portland bedroom with her family at her side, she took the prescribed fatal dose of barbiturates.

As mentioned above, taking one's own life is not illegal, but assisting another to commit suicide is. Medical aid in dying (MAID) laws have been enacted in some areas of the country, providing an exception to this ban.[8] As of the fall of 2019, MAID is legally available in nine states (California, Colorado, Hawaii, Maine, Montana, New Jersey, Oregon, Vermont, and Washington) and the District of Columbia; legislative, judicial, and administrative actions and challenges are ongoing, not only in these states but throughout the nation. MAID is also legal throughout Canada and in several European countries. The state of Oregon has the longest American experience, dating back to 1997, so I will use the regulations and practice established there as definition and illustration. The Oregon Death with Dignity statute defines MAID as a process in which a terminally ill patient receives "a prescription for medication to end his or her life in a humane and dignified manner."[9] Oregon physicians are required to report details of patients who die from MAID, so reliable data on its use and outcomes are readily and publicly available. As of the most recent report (February 2019), a total of 1,459 known Oregonians have died from ingesting a lethal dose of medication. In 2017, 259 individuals received prescriptions for fatal medication and at least 157 people died from taking it (more than 35,000 people died in Oregon that year, making MAID responsible for 0.4% of deaths).[10]

The Oregon law requires that for a patient to receive aid in dying, they must be at least eighteen years of age and a resident of the state of Oregon, be capable of making and communicating their own health care decisions, and be diagnosed with a terminal illness that will likely lead to death within six months. They must also be capable of swallowing the fatal dose (or injecting it into a feeding tube) by themselves. They must verbally request assisted dying to their attending physician twice, at least fifteen days apart, and also provide that doctor with a signed and witnessed written request. They are required to consult another physician to confirm the terminal state and diagnosis as well as their ability to make their own medical decisions. If either of these doctors suspects underlying depression or mental illness is impacting the patient's rational ability, a psychology or psychiatry evaluation is needed (this was done for three patients who died in 2018). Note that at no time is the patient required to justify their request based on extent of symptoms or other description of their suffering. The attending physician must also advise the patient to inform their next of kin of their plans, to not ingest the deadly dose in public, and that they may opt out at any time and for any reason. Opting out is not uncommon; at least a third of patients who receive a lethal prescription do not use it.

The major arguments for further legalization of MAID center on its role as an option for those experiencing intractable symptoms. But this is not the most common reason people choose MAID. Inadequate pain control or the fear of it is given as a reason only by about one in four who die this way.[11] By far the most potent and frequent concerns leading to MAID are fear of the loss of autonomy and of the ability to engage in activities that make life enjoyable, with nearly nine out of ten identifying both of these as reasons for their request. Loss of dignity is also a large concern, cited by about three out of four. These reasons correlate with the underlying diagnoses of those who choose this path. The most common diagnosis for patients who choose MAID is cancer, accounting for 76 percent of Oregonians who have used this practice. As a contrast, while about 22 percent of Americans die from cancer and 23 percent from heart disease, less than 5 percent of those dying by MAID have terminal cardiac disease. This fits with the clinical courses of these illnesses; patients with cancer commonly experience a progressive and inexorable increase in symptoms and decline in function—that is, they and their doctors can recognize their impending demise. Contrarily, the course for those with heart disease is characterized by cyclic exacerbations and recoveries, and many patients die suddenly. Consequently, fewer patients with heart disease are likely to recognize their terminal state and initiate the MAID request process.

Of particular interest regarding the reasons for choosing MAID is the example of amyotrophic lateral sclerosis (ALS, Lou Gehrig's disease). In the general population, this disease accounts for about 0.002 percent of deaths, yet 8 percent of those who receive MAID in Oregon have that disease. ALS is the exemplar of my nurse friend's "garage diagnoses," causing those it afflicts to lose motor function and the ability to walk, work, speak, eat, and control elimination on a year by year, month by month, sometimes day by day basis, while usually keeping the ability to think, reason, and feel totally intact. This results in the nightmarish situation of being alert and aware, feeling every pain, sensing every emotion, noticing every person who avoids looking at you, and being unable to communicate or respond. While, for the few fortunate patients with a more gradual course, assistive devices can provide mobility and the ability to communicate, the eventual result for all is loss of ability to swallow and breathe. Feeding tubes and mechanical ventilators can keep the body functioning for months or years, but many patients, anticipating this type of existence, choose to exert their integrity and achieve victory in the only effective way left to them. They can choose the moment, ambience, and companions for their death. They may see this act as a way of preventing the oppressing disease of robbing them further. In this way, dying can be a victory over the disease.

Ethicists are divided, as is the public, on the question of whether MAID constitutes a moral act. Arguments against it include those of sanctity of life, the character of medical practice as a healing art, and the risk of the "slippery slope." This latter issue raises concern that acceptance of MAID might lead to other practices, like voluntary euthanasia (discussed below) or even involuntary euthanasia of the elderly, demented, feeble, or others seen as somehow "less than persons." Arguments supporting MAID center on relief of suffering and the self-determination and autonomy of human persons, on a person's right to decide when and under what circumstances life is no longer desired. The current trends are that more and more Americans believe that this should be a legal option, and it is expected that it will become available in more jurisdictions in the coming years. The members of the baby boom generation, those born between 1946 and 1964, seem to particularly value control of their own destiny. We will look further at the issue of autonomy in chapter 5.

As already stated, MAID, as currently practiced in the United States, requires that the patient be both mentally and psychologically able to request the prescription and physically capable of taking it. In addition, for someone to obtain the lethal prescription, they must already be dying from some other cause. The argument has been made that this creates a "right" for these qualified patients that is not available to the infirm, demented, and those living with suffering but not in the terminal stages of an illness. The counterargument is that this is not discrimination; it is protection. The statutes as currently written do not allow for anyone except the patient to decide, in real time, the time when life should end. An issue that produces de facto discrimination in the availability of MAID is the cost of the medications. The cost of a lethal dose of secobarbital, the preferred drug, rose by more than

700 percent between 2010 and 2016, from about \$387 to \$2,878.[12] The cost of the medication is almost invariably borne by the patient. The costs as well as shortages of this drug have caused prescribing physicians to improvise, usually using selected medicine combinations. Another practical matter is that every state that has legalized MAID limits its availability to legal residents of that state. Residents of states without legal aid in dying are not able to participate. This is why Brittany Maynard had to move to and establish legal residency in Oregon before obtaining MAID. At this time, the only place in the world where MAID is practiced that allows noncitizens to participate is Switzerland.

Voluntary Euthanasia

As MAID requires both mental and physical competence to request and self-administer the lethal prescription, patients often elect it based on fear of what is likely to happen in the future rather than what is occurring at the present. Those who seek MAID might therefore sacrifice days or weeks of life knowing that if they wait too long to ingest the lethal dose, they could lose the capability of doing so. One option for ending life that is not legally available anywhere in the United States is voluntary euthanasia, the ending of a person's life at their request, usually by a lethal injection by a physician. (In the United States we do, however, practice involuntary euthanasia, calling it capital punishment.) Voluntary euthanasia is currently legal in the Netherlands, Belgium, and Luxembourg. Laws in these nations limit the availability of this procedure to their own citizens.

After a ruling by the Dutch Supreme Court in the 1980s, physicians in the Netherlands who aided in the voluntary and requested death of a patient were deemed immune from criminal prosecution, providing they did so with what the court termed "due care." This aid could mean either providing a lethal prescription (like MAID in the United States) or directly administering a fatal injection. Euthanasia was formally legalized in Holland in 2002, giving the Dutch now more than three decades of informative experience. In 2014, 5,306 people died from MAID and euthanasia in Holland (3.8% of total deaths).[13] Euthanasia may only be performed if the patient requests it; a pro-euthanasia advance directive can serve as that legal request for patients no longer able to speak for themselves, but physicians have been reluctant to act with only that authorization. The Dutch Termination of Life on Request and Assisted Suicide Act established six criteria for "due care," all of which a physician must comply with in order to be practicing within the law:[14] (1) The physician must be convinced that the patient's request is voluntary and well considered. (2) The physician must be convinced that the patient's suffering is unbearable and without prospect of relief. (3) The patient must be informed about their situation and prospects. (4) The physician and the patient together must be convinced that there is no reasonable alternative for the situation. (5) At least one other independent physician must be consulted. (6) The ending of life must be performed in a professionally careful way. The physician is required to report each case to a regional review committee, which weighs whether the legal conditions have been met. Note that there is no requirement for the presence of a terminal disease for someone to receive assistance in dying in Holland; relief of unbearable suffering is the focus and goal.

As with the Oregon experience with MAID, the Dutch data shed light on the motivations of people who choose euthanasia. Most Dutch patients receiving aid in dying or euthanasia have underlying cancer; the second most common diagnoses are neurologic diseases. In a study of deaths of patients with terminal cancer in the Utrecht area, there was no difference in the presence of either intractable symptoms or unbearable suffering between patients who eventually died with or without euthanasia.[15] The only differences the investigators found between the two groups were that those who received euthanasia were more highly educated and had more frequently completed a pro-euthanasia advance directive. Again, the driving forces appear to be autonomy, choice, control, and fear.

Ethical issues that remain unsettled in these European nations include questions of if or when aided death can be provided to a patient who is not able to competently request it at that point. The issue of advance directives was mentioned above, but the rights of other groups remain controversial. Are severely deformed or terminally ill infants and children allowed to receive euthanasia with their parents' consent? Can a legal surrogate for a patient with terminal dementia request the ending of that person's life? Can patients suffering from severe psychiatric illness obtain relief by requesting the end of their life? Several of these scenarios raise the question as to whether the euthanasia would be truly voluntary. For populations only a few generations removed from the atrocities of the Holocaust, those are active and relevant considerations.

In the United States, surveys generally reveal more public support for MAID and even voluntary euthanasia than would be suggested by the small number of jurisdictions in which MAID legalization has occurred. An intriguing survey of health care personnel at Yale–New Haven Hospital (in a state where MAID is illegal) lends insight into current opinions.[16] The participants in the study were provided a scenario of an elderly, bedridden, terminally ill patient with cancer who has at most six months to live, is in pain, and wishes to end his life with the assistance of his physician. They were then given three variations of the story to consider: in the first, the patient was mentally competent, able to take the lethal medications, and requested MAID; in the second, the patient was competent but unable to take the drugs and was requesting euthanasia; and in the third, the patient was not competent but had requested euthanasia in his advance directive and his DPAH concurred in requesting it. About two-thirds of the respondents (about half of whom were physicians) thought that for this patient, MAID was ethical and should be a legal option. More than half supported the morality of voluntary euthanasia for the competent patient and said it should be legalized. A bit surprisingly, the number who supported euthanasia requested by the advance directive and DPAH was higher than those who supported euthanasia for the competent patient, nearly as many as supported MAID. Whether the findings of this single institution study are representative of more generalized attitudes is unclear, but this report strongly suggests that, in the United States, we are only beginning a protracted process of debate, experimentation, legislation, and litigation about the rights of terminally ill persons to choose the time and mode of their death.

BOB AND DR. FREUD

Sigmund Freud first noted symptoms of oral cancer, undoubtedly related to his ever-burning cigars, when he was sixty-six.[17] Over the next sixteen years he underwent numerous surgeries and courses of primitive radiation treatment while continuing his extraordinary scholarship and practice. Over the last years of his life, he gave his primary physician two explicit charges: that the relationship between the two of them must be characterized by "open, unalloyed truth" and that "when the time comes, you won't let me suffer unnecessarily." As the cancer inexorably progressed, as he reached the end of his life, an existence which had become for him "a little island of pain floating on a sea of indifference," he reminded his doctor of their covenants. Repeated doses of morphine allowed Dr. Freud to fall into a sleep from which he never awakened.

I believe Bob also hoped for the end of his life to be sleep without awakening, the "sweet peace" that Freud had asked for eighty years previously. He had made the same requests of me that Sigmund Freud had of his doctor: honesty and relief. Bob was able to identify the things that gave his life meaning and also recognized that there would come a time when the depth of his suffering overwhelmed that meaning. Together we planned for that time; when he requested it, I would initiate an infusion of midazolam, titrate the dosage to achieve palliative sedation, and continue it until he died. We missed one item in our plan, though; we neglected to consider the precept attributed to E. A. Murphy, that if there is a chance of something going wrong, it will. When Bob recognized that the scales had tipped the other way, that there was only suffering left, I was away on vacation. Communication snafus, difficulty locating my documentation, and conflicts between the covering physician and an insistent family friend all conspired such that palliative sedation was not initiated. I realize that, just as I recommend patients to have advance directives to be sure their wishes are carried out, I should have made an advance plan that could be implemented if I were unavailable so that my promise could be kept. Fortunately, the interventions that were prescribed for Bob did provide some sedation and relief, and this final phase went very quickly, so he did slip from this life apparently at peace.

5

IT'S MY LIFE, ISN'T IT?

By what right, with what motive could anyone presume to dispute my right to dispose of these two–three weeks of my term? Whose business is it to judge?
—Fyodor Dostoevsky, *The Idiot*

In 1963, Lesley Gore hit number one on the pop charts with a song proclaiming that since it was her party, she'd cry if she wanted to. The topic of that song was disappointed love, but it expressed a clear assertion: what I own is mine to do with as I choose. In ethical parlance, the term applied to this claim is "autonomy," the ability of a free individual to make decisions free of coercion. This idea is consistent with the American cultural heritage metaphors of "life, liberty, and the pursuit of happiness" and the "frontier pioneer spirit." Most Americans would answer the question posed by the title of this chapter with "of course it is."

Lesley Gore's proclamation about her right to cry is followed by an expansion of her premise; she sees her action not only as her right but also as a reasonable response to what she has endured. The next lyrics claim anyone would cry in a similar situation. In patient care arenas, this attitude gets expressed in phrases like "If this were my mother, I would never put her through this" or "I can't imagine what I would do if this were me." When we know or hear of people facing life-and-death choices, especially in the face of intolerable suffering or indignity, we experience an empathic emotional response that may lead to a rational consideration of what we might desire to happen if we were in a similar situation. We do well to pay attention to those feelings and thoughts when they arise and allow them to inform the choices we will have to make for ourselves and likely also for some of those close to us.

The right of autonomy, of personal liberty, is not absolute. We understand that our freedom to act independently in society encounters limits when our actions affect others or violate legal prohibitions. But in the world of medicine and life-and-death decisions, what constraints are there on our autonomy? Is it really my life? The obvious and simple answer is "yes," after all, whose else could it be? But is it really that simple and obvious?

AUTONOMY AND BIOETHICS

The roots of American bioethics extend throughout Western philosophical and religious thought. We have already encountered several moral principles, including those of substituted judgment, double effect, and confidentiality. There are four principles, though, that are often cited as the tetrad of pillars upholding bioethical thought and decision making in the United States. In particular cases or scenarios, these tenets may agree or conflict with each other, but the questions they ask should always be addressed when searching for guidance in right behavior. This quartet consists of beneficence, nonmaleficence, justice, and autonomy.

Beneficence means that the practitioner must act with the good of the patient as the primary goal. The oath attributed to Hippocrates includes the line, "Whatever houses I may visit, I will come for the benefit of the sick." The confidence that a physician is acting with the patient's interest preeminent is essential for a therapeutic relationship. The idea that a physician would allow financial gain, scientific prestige, or personal prejudice to displace the primacy of patient benefit is repugnant. Populations who have endured long-term prejudice and disadvantage may have difficulty reaching a trusting relationship with a physician or with the medical system; their care providers may find that trust needs to be earned on an individual basis. More recently, physician productivity requirements, performance and outcomes payment systems, and the increasing bottom-line focus of health care systems risk damaging this essential character of the healing relationship. Despite these pressures, though, it remains a tenet of American medicine that when I, as a patient, receive medical care, it must be provided with my benefit foremost in mind.

Nonmaleficence is the countervalue to beneficence and says that harm to the patient must be avoided or minimized. Probably the most famous phrase that Hippocrates never uttered (not even in Greek) is *primum non nocere*, Latin for "first, do no harm." The source of this mandate is obscure, but its pithiness perfectly conveys the concept of nonmaleficence, the avoidance of causing injury. The simplest example of a conflict between nonmaleficence and beneficence is that of a surgical procedure. The surgeon perpetrates injury by cutting into a patient, but the intended good, cure of disease or alleviation of symptoms, is positive and likely enough to justify the harm inflicted. In other medical situations, unintended harms, even serious or fatal injuries, may develop, like medication side effects or hospital complications. Damage may not be purely physical but psychological (body image), social (impotence), or financial. In weighing medical decisions, the beneficence/nonmaleficence equation is usually presented in terms of risks and benefits and most of the time is straightforward. As we have seen, though, when it comes to judgments that arise at the end of life, this equation is less easily solved.

As most commonly stated, the principle of justice seeks equal opportunity and fair distribution. Recent and current political arguments over US health care delivery blare the fact that our medical insurance and payment structure is far from equitable and raise the question as to whether the American public actually desires a just system. Even though it is clear that access to health care, especially expensive procedures and medications, is strongly related to socioeconomic status, the question of social justice is rarely raised in American medicine, as it raises the specters of health care rationing or further governmental intervention. Patients raise the justice question in one of two ways. I have heard many claim, "I paid into this system all my life, and I deserve to get whatever I want out of it." Alternatively, a more altruistic approach is exemplified by someone who expresses that limited resources should go to someone younger, an ill child, for example. Within families, the dying elder may choose to forego expensive interventions with the idea that their wealth could be better spent on their children or by a charitable cause.

The concept of human autonomy states that each person is able to function independently without control by others and is often described with words like "independence" and "self-determination." In the medical realm, autonomy is manifested by the concept that an individual has the right to accept or decline any medical intervention or procedure. Violation of this right is grounds for possible civil or even criminal penalties. As discussed in chapter 2, autonomy has traditionally been viewed as a negative right, the authority to refuse whatever may be proposed. More recently, though, especially with the increasing availability of medical aid in dying, a positive or imperative aspect has been claimed, the ability to "die when and how I want to."

While ethical judgments should be influenced by all four of these basic principles, current practice tends to emphasize patient autonomy as preeminent among the foursome. This is largely a rejection of the paternalistic, authoritarian role that physicians took on in the past. The preeminence of autonomy is exemplified when a patient with a serious acute medical problem refuses treatment, even if it is clear that the likely outcome will be worsening of the condition, increasing symptoms, and more aggressive and costly treatment when they reach the stage of desperation and then demand therapy. My colleagues, especially those in social work, put it this way: "People have the right to make bad decisions."

LEGAL AUTONOMY IN THE UNITED STATES

The legal right for self-determination, the right to refuse any medical intervention, is well established, and the right of a designated legal surrogate to speak for the patient who cannot speak for themselves is guaranteed. The basis for the validity of surrogate decision making, substituted judgment, is the idea that the surrogate should know best what the patient would say if they were able to do so. The breadth of that right has been legally determined in two major court cases.

In 1976, the parents of Karen Ann Quinlan, a young woman who had fallen into an irreversible coma after ingesting diazepam and alcohol and relied on a ventilator machine to keep her alive because she couldn't breathe on her own, sued her physicians because they refused to remove the ventilator. They argued that Karen would not want this treatment to continue and claimed authority to speak for her. The New Jersey Supreme Court ruled that Karen's right to refuse life-sustaining treatment, to be disconnected from the ventilator, was still valid even though she could not express her refusal herself. At the same time, the court provided legal immunity to physicians who withheld or withdrew such treatments based on advance directives and surrogate requests. The case also encouraged states to enact "living will" statutes so that individuals could legally document their wishes and those wishes would be carried out.

While the Quinlan decision was technically authoritative only for the state of New Jersey, in 1990, the US Supreme Court heard the case of Nancy Cruzan, a young woman from Missouri who, because of an accident, remained in a persistent vegetative state. Nancy was not on a ventilator; she was breathing on her own, but her body was maintained by feedings through a tube surgically implanted into her stomach. Her parents had filed suit, stating that she would not have wanted this treatment, and asked that the feedings be stopped and the tube removed. The court found that there was no legal distinction between a ventilator and a tube feeding system as far as being a life-sustaining medical procedure and allowed the family's demands to be acceded to. This set precedent for the entire nation, and now all states recognize the right of a patient to name a surrogate, a durable power of attorney for health care, to speak for them if they cannot speak for themselves.

The principles and precedents of the Quinlan and Cruzan cases are now widely accepted and espoused in the medical and legal communities, but that does not mean that they are always followed. Doctors often feel more comfortable not starting an intervention like a breathing machine than they do stopping it. Withholding it feels more like allowing nature to take its course, while withdrawing it feels more like killing. Governmental and ethical authorities are clear that withholding and withdrawing are legally and morally equivalent. But to the one who actually turns off the machine and removes the breathing tube, it may not feel that way.

Another scenario that may negate a patient's wishes to discontinue treatment, especially artificial nutrition and hydration, is that of institutional policy. Some long-term care facilities, because of "pro-life" religious underpinnings or fear of lawsuit, prohibit stopping tube feedings or other life-supporting care they consider "ordinary." I have cared for several patients who were transferred to our inpatient hospice unit simply to have a feeding tube withdrawn. Unfortunately, most of the time they were not allowed back into their "home" facilities and died separated from those who had cared for and about them previously.

CLAIMS ON OUR AUTONOMY: LEGITIMATE AND ILLICIT

When Brittany Maynard, the young woman with glioblastoma we met in the last chapter, chose to end her life, she was asserting her autonomy—that her body, her life, was her own. She put it this way: "I do not want to die. But I am dying. And I want to die on my own terms."[1] She made her story public in part, in collaboration with the advocacy organization Compassion and Choices, to fight for the availability of medical aid in dying (MAID). Responses to Brittany's very public statements and death were wide-ranging. Some applauded her courage, but others claimed she had allowed herself to be a prop in a publicity stunt. This criticism was particularly made by those identifying as "pro-life." As I reviewed these responses in writing this chapter, I found those posts from people who had similar diseases and were facing their own demise particularly poignant. One example is that of Philip G. Johnson, a US Navy veteran with a grade 3 astrocytoma who was then in seminary training to become a Catholic priest, who said that he saw Brittany's decision as "anything but brave." His view was that making the choice to die "on her own terms" robbed her of the chance to be cared for by family during her terminal suffering, something he envisioned as an intimate and loving gift.[2] Maggie Karner, who spent much of her life working with international medical mission teams and also identified herself as "pro-life" also had developed glioblastoma multiforme. She saw sanctity and value in life, no matter how her body and mind were assaulted by the disease. She then reflected on the quality of the life of her own father, who was quadriplegic, and wondered whether Brittany would have seen such life as "useless."[3]

As I read these and many other posts from that time, I was impressed by the kind and caring feelings behind these disapproving statements but also by the fact that most of the moral critics seemed to be saying that Brittany Maynard's "own terms" for dying were mistaken, unjustified, or even evil and that their personal "own terms" were right. Years of medical practice have taught me that the only person who can define their "own terms" for valuing life is the person who is living that life. The only one who can negotiate their way through suffering and death is the one enduring that suffering and dying that death. I may, with all sense of well-meaning, offer my concern and even express disagreement, but it is hubris to think that somehow I have a better understanding of how that person feels and what that person fears than they do. I have not had their life experience, I have not walked a mile in their moccasins, and I have no claim on their life or death. If I exploit that person's story, suffering, or dying to promote my own thoughts, positions, or political agenda, I do so at my peril. We will return to this idea in a couple pages when we review another public case, that of Terri Schiavo.

There are those, however, with legitimate claims on our lives and deaths. The first claimant is fate, luck, serendipity, whatever one chooses to call the unpredictability of life. The coronary blood clot, the cancer growing somewhere inside, the texting driver, the stray bullet, even our advancing age do not submit to our autonomy. The choices we have available are only those we can make in response to such events. This point may seem obvious, but in my experience working with the dying, a frequent obstacle to cogent decision making is resentment or anger at the apparent randomness and injustice of death and terminal illness. We expect life to be fair and struggle to make sense of it or find meaning when it doesn't seem to be that way. This struggle has been ongoing since antiquity with proposed solutions widely varied, such as the will of God, karma, or, "hey, stuff happens." We will think about this more in chapter 9 when we explore issues of meaning.

There is another whose opinion and agenda do matter, do have influence on one's choices in life and death, and that is the state. Governments can and do claim suzerainty in issues of dying. In military action and criminal sentencing, the state can even mandate death. Governments keep track of births and deaths and prosecute unlawful taking of life. This is where Brittany Maynard found a roadblock, with the claims of the state of California outweighing her own autonomy. She desired an option available in some jurisdictions but not in others, and she and her family made major life changes to be in compliance with statutes and regulations so that she could achieve her goals.

Voluntary Cession of Life Ownership

One night, while we were having dinner at a Chinese restaurant, I started up a conversation with my wife, Pat, about MAID. It had been some time since we had discussed this topic; I expected to hear what had been her personal position in the past, that since God alone is the source of life, God alone has authority to take life. She surprised me, though, when she said that she had come to realize that there are situations in which death may be preferable to continued life. But when the topic changed to the hypothetical possibility of me choosing to end my life that way, she strongly objected. She said, "I remember that day when we had Smokie [our elkhound] put to sleep; it was the most horrible moment in my life. I wanted to say 'good-bye' again, but it was already over, and there was no going back. If that was you, I don't know if I could endure it." Even though I'd thought about this issue for a long time, including whether I would choose that option if it were available, I had simply not adequately considered its effect on the one I love. My dying, my suffering, would end at the moment of my death, but her pain would go on. This illustrated clearly for me the fact that when we engage in the process of loving and being loved, when we enter into a committed relationship, we relinquish at least a bit of our independent control over our own selves. The Hebrew scriptures term this process becoming "one flesh."[4]

In American romantic parlance, we talk about "giving" ourselves to the one we love. In popular media and culture, this is usually a reference to sexual union, but in reality the "gift" is much more complete and profound. When I gave my love and my self to Pat, and she gave hers to me, we both abrogated some of our own independence and autonomy. If a child enters such a relationship, yet another lays strong claim to our life. We deny our own whims because the claim of this new totally dependent other must take precedence. For most people, it is exactly these and other intimate relationships that give great joy and meaning to life. But when we approach our own death, these others are the ones who will be most affected by our leaving. The claim that their suffering and grieving makes on our autonomy cannot be dismissed lightly.

Every person voluntarily cedes some ownership of their life to others, as Pat and I have to each other. There are, of course, many personal relationships other than the spousal and parental ones that can make these demands; each reader can quickly imagine who those are in their own lives. In my oncology practice, I occasionally saw this cession played out with unfortunate consequences. Many an elderly patient with advanced cancer told me confidentially that they did not desire to receive further chemotherapy but that they chose to continue it for someone else, usually a child. Not only were these parents taking on the burden of putting up with side effects of treatment, they were also ceding their autonomy over their own life and death. Sometimes these were loving gifts, sometimes they were evidence of poor communication and dysfunctional relationships, but in each case, the patient made a choice about living and dying that acknowledged the claim of another. Unfortunately, often these treatments did not work out, so neither the patient nor family received what they thought they wanted.

In addition to other individuals, people often "give their lives" to causes or philosophies. For example, for someone who has dedicated extensive energy to a charitable organization, wondering what will happen to that group after they die is, in a way, recognition of a claim on their own life and death. An even more common cession is seen in those who choose to commit themselves to a religion or deity.

One religious creed, the *Brief Statement of Faith* of the Presbyterian Church, begins, "In life and in death we belong to God."[5] While this phrase can be interpreted in many ways, it illustrates a common religious concept—that the creative divine being demands submission from the creation. One who believes in a God who generates and sustains life, who remains involved in the world, must recognize one's own obligation to accede to (or possibly rebel from) that God. In the next chapter we will try to further flesh out how the relationships between personal spirituality or religion and end-of-life choices play out in practice. Even those who reject the idea of a creator live attached to some underlying principles, though those may evolve through the course of their lives. Those underlying allegiances might be as mundane as being a rabid member of the Cleveland Browns Dawg Pound or as noble as Mother Teresa's care of the dying destitute in Kolkata.

Individual life principles vary widely, from greed to gratitude, power to philanthropy, fashion to family, jealousy to justice, lechery to love. These things that we devote pieces of our lives to are exactly those "terms" we talk about when we say we want to die "on our own terms." They are our own expressions of autonomy as well as the terms of our surrender. If we are to die with dignity, we must die with integrity, consonant with the values of our lives, respecting the cessions we have made and affirming our autonomy simultaneously.

WHEN THINGS GO WRONG: TERRI AND THE CIRCUS

On February 20, 1990, when Brittany Maynard was five years old, a twenty-six-year-old Florida woman named Theresa Marie Schiavo suffered a cardiac arrest, possibly from a severe chemical imbalance brought on by an eating disorder.[6] Terri, as she was known, suffered devastating brain damage resulting in a persistent vegetative state (PVS). In this condition, the primitive brain functions that keep the heart beating, the lungs breathing, and the body's waking and sleeping cycles remain intact, but all higher functions are lost. The cerebral cortex, the part of the brain that makes us a person, is dead. In other words, patients in PVS have no ability to feel pain or experience love; they do not get hungry or feel full; and they cannot taste, see, hear, smell, or touch. They are unable to be happy because of a lover's presence or feel embarrassment because their diaper is dirty. The term "vegetative" is used because there is no ability for any purposeful action. Even the abilities of lower animals—that of a cat to bask in the sun, a fish to flop on a hook, or an ant to find a crumb at a picnic—are gone. Many describe these patients as a body that remains present even after the person who inhabited it has departed.

Since these patients' bodies go through sleeping and waking cycles, sometimes it looks like "there's somebody in there." This can be very perplexing as well as emotionally wrenching to loved ones who are present. Terri Schiavo's husband, Michael, and her parents, Robert and Mary Schindler, watched this as it went on for years. Terri's bodily functions were otherwise intact; she was breathing on her own, her heart was strong, and her vital órgans worked well. Her body required only food and water to continue surviving, and this was provided by a tube surgically placed into her stomach (PEG). About four months after her cardiac arrest, Terri's husband, Michael, was appointed as her guardian. Terri spent the ensuing fifteen years until her death being cared for in nursing homes and had no improvement in her neurologic status. Stating that he believed she would not want to be kept alive in this condition, Michael filed a petition in 1998 to have the feeding tube removed from Terri's body.

Terri's parents opposed Michael's request to remove the tube and filed a court action to prevent it. Their raised concern was that Terri (and therefore Michael) had been awarded a malpractice settlement, which, along with the fact that Michael was now involved with another woman, made his ability to objectively speak for Terri questionable. Twenty months later the County Circuit Court judge ruled that Terri would have chosen to have the PEG removed and ordered that it be done. The parents appealed, and the case proceeded up through the court system. In April 2001, eleven years after the initial event, the PEG was taken out. The parents immediately filed a motion claiming that Michael had committed perjury, and the tube was ordered reinserted two days after it had been removed. Over the ensuing two and a half years, multiple other physicians examined Ms. Schiavo at court order, and at least five courts either affirmed the original decision or declined to review the case, all in concurrence with the finding that Terri would want the tube out. The parents then filed a federal lawsuit, and Florida governor Jeb Bush issued a legal brief in support of them. The Federal District Court ruled that it lacked jurisdiction, and on October 15, 2003, the PEG was removed for the second time. Six days later, in an attempt to counter this action, the Florida legislature enacted "Terri's Law" enabling the governor to grant a "one-time stay" in certain cases. Governor Bush issued such an executive order, and the feeding tube was reinserted. He also ordered the appointment of a new guardian *ad litem*, someone who would investigate independently to determine what is in the person's best interest. This expert agreed that Terri was indeed in a persistent vegetative state with no chance of improvement. The next year the Florida Supreme Court declared "Terri's Law" unconstitutional; Governor Bush requested review by the US Supreme Court, but this was declined. On March 18, 2005, the tube was removed for the third time. On that same date, to take up Terri's by now highly publicized case, the US Congress, which had been on Easter recess, reconvened and President George W. Bush flew back to Washington. A circus-like frenzy ensued in which multiple physician members of Congress watched grainy videotapes, held up brain scans in Congress, and then made varying claims about the accuracy of the diagnosis of persistent vegetative state. The House of Representatives issued subpoenas for Michael Schiavo, physicians and hospital personnel, and, remarkably, Terri herself. President Bush signed legislation passed by Congress granting federal courts the power to review the case. The parents filed a motion for such a review and asked the federal district court to order reinsertion of the tube. All courts, including the Supreme Court, denied this motion. Theresa Schiavo died on March 31, 2005, thirteen days after the tube was removed for the final time.

Fortunately, cases such as Terri Schiavo's are aberrant. As the events around her death illustrate, legislatures, courts, and executive governmental offices are poor venues for decisions regarding individual end-of-life actions. As we have mentioned repeatedly, governing authorities have enacted and supported advance directive statutes and procedures in order to keep them from the necessity of exerting their power, and usually those processes work reasonably well.

Terri's story, like that of Brittany Maynard and virtually every other dying person, illustrates the fact that one's life is neither lived nor ended in a vacuum. Apart from the circumstances over which we have no control, none of these other claims on our lives need determine our choices about our departure, but they must be accounted for in our deliberation for those choices to be authentic and responsible. Again, these are "our own terms" for our dying. Yes, we "own" our lives. The intentional ending of one's own life may be an act of integrity, love, and wholeness, but the idea that it is a "victimless" act is folly. A death with dignity must be a death with integrity and wholeness, not one of selfishness and isolation.

6

WHAT'S GOD GOT TO DO WITH IT?

An' the Gobble-uns 'll git you Ef you Don't Watch Out!
—James Whitcomb Riley, *Little Orphant Annie*

Like millions of other kids, I knelt by my bed and prayed, "Now I lay me down to sleep, I pray the Lord my soul to keep; if I should die before I wake, I pray the Lord my soul to take." As a little child, I may not have understood much of what death was all about, but this prayer impressed on me that it was serious business, and, like Little Orphant Annie's Gobble-uns, or the monsters living under my bed, it could strike at any time. It might happen if I didn't watch out!

Humans fear that which is unknown or threatening, and most of us, if we think about our deaths at all, experience a sense of dread. This is one reason I advocate looking at our own dying with as much realism and honesty as we can muster. While we are healthy, we usually consider our demise as an abstract concept, keeping what is fearful at arm's length. But becoming acquainted with death can be useful as a way of spying out the strengths and strategies of an enemy we know we will face some day. Or perhaps it is a pathway to get to know a future friend.

We deal with our fear of dying in a variety of ways. Children try not to think about it because, for five- to ten-year-olds, thinking about it might make it happen, and if they don't think or talk about it, it might not occur. This magical ideation frequently persists into adulthood; many deal with disturbing ideas by banishing them from their minds, saying, like Scarlett O'Hara, "I'll think about that tomorrow." Some take a military approach, fighting off what is feared; delving into the details of disease, treatments, and options; looking for yet another way to try to "beat it." Many, when facing death, turn to religion, to questions of meaning, afterlife, judgment, or reward to come. All of these, as well as other approaches and combinations thereof, are attempts to find hope or discover significance.

So, if we dread our dying, what exactly is it that we are afraid of? In my experience, most people's forebodings fit into one of three basic anxieties. First is the fear of what dying will be like: Will it take very long? What will I do when I can't get around anymore? Will I have to let my son change my dirty diaper? Will I be in pain? Short of breath? Anxious, agitated, or delirious? Will I whimper or scream and make a fool of myself? Will I stink? Second is the fear of loss: What will happen to my children if I'm not there for them? What stories will they tell about me after I'm gone? Will I look sick so that no one wants to visit me? Will I be one of those people that others look away from? What if nobody wants to listen to what I really want to say? Finally, there is the fear of the unknowable: Have I been good enough? Did I believe in the right things? What truly happens when we die? What if there really is nothing else except this? What did I do that was worthwhile? Will my death matter? Did it even matter at all that I was alive? Will I be forgotten?

EMILY, CHARLENE, AND GOD

Emily knew that Charlene would live. It was guaranteed; it was there in black and white. Her Baptist upbringing had taught her that what was written in the Bible could be relied on. Jesus had promised, "So I tell you, whatever you ask for in prayer, believe that you have received it, and it will be yours."[1]

It had worked before. On several occasions she had personally experienced divine presence, so she knew that God existed, that God cared. When she prayed, she sensed a tangible presence and power that was available to her. Things she had prayed about seemed to work out the way she thought they should. She could attest to the truth of the verse from the New Testament book of James, "The prayer of the righteous is powerful and effective."[2]

Charlene had acute leukemia. It wasn't fair. Charlene was beautiful, young, vibrant, and sure of the grace of God in her life. She was a good friend, one of Emily's intimate circle. Emily's distress when she thought about her friend withering in that big city hospital bed was nearly paralyzing. The only energy she could generate was in harnessing those wrenching emotions, yoking them with the prayers she made. Her instructions were also from James: "Are any among you sick? . . . pray for them." The passage included a clear expected outcome: "Prayer . . . will save the sick, and the Lord will raise them up."[3] Emily wasn't naïve enough to think it was likely that a miraculous immediate cure was likely, but she knew that, whatever treatment Charlene would have to endure, whatever complications would develop, however long it took, the outcome was assured: Charlene would get well. Charlene would live.

But it didn't work out that way. During the final few days of Charlene's life, Emily sat by the bed, holding her friend's skeletal hand, the hand of a body that was rapidly failing, the hand of a friend who, at times, could barely speak because of medication effects and worsening weakness. Emily, the persistent prayer warrior, wielded every weapon she knew, fended off doubt, harnessed the infinity of divine power to produce what would now be a dramatic miracle. She was both anxious and excited about what she was experiencing. The time was clearly short; it would need to come about soon. She repeated her mantra: "The Bible says it; I believe it; the healing will appear." But, like Jesus, the one she trusted, Charlene suffered, Charlene died, and Charlene was buried.

Emily knew those scriptural passages read so often at funerals, reassurances like "I am the resurrection and the life. Those who believe in me, even though they die, will live,"[4] but, as she sat through the memorial service the words were hollow, meaningless, irrelevant. Even worse were the clichés intended to comfort: "God must have a good reason for taking such a lovely girl." "You know, all things work together for good." "Charlene is happy in the arms of Jesus." "Think about all the wonderful times you had together." "She is not suffering anymore."

Emily had been so certain. The well-meaning people who tried to console her with these platitudes, many of them the same ones who had assured her that God could be trusted to keep promises, couldn't see that Charlene's death violated everything they had taught her. Here, now, when it really mattered, it turned out to be a crock. And if this part of what she had learned in church wasn't reliable, then what else wasn't true? Should she just abandon the whole thing? She still thought that God existed—she had experienced this for herself—but how did that really matter? The universe didn't work the way she thought it should. Her world was disrupted and uncertain. She would have to find her own way.

Emily buried herself in her journalism studies and career. She was good at it and attained some success. To all appearances she was the achiever, the accomplished young woman all had expected her to become. But in the dark and swampy places deep inside, she struggled for reliable footing, searched for a glimmer of direction.

The first flicker emerged in an unlikely place. She began to volunteer at a local hospice agency. Here she encountered people asking the same questions she posed, working through the same grief she suffered. They, like her, found few answers, but now at least she knew she was not alone. Charlene's death still did not make sense, and she realized that it never would. She began to comprehend that the divine could not be found in the pat explanations she had learned. There was no need for God if there was no doubt. She began to find the transcendent in the questions, the paradoxes, the uncertainty. Emily followed her quest into this unsettled territory, a quest that eventually led to seminary training. She now serves as director of chaplaincy services at a large medical center. By taking her faith journey seriously, by challenging what didn't work, by getting comfortable with uncertainty, she found the peace that rote answers could never provide. Wrestling in her woundedness had provided strength, insight, and compassion, the vital resources for her therapeutic presence with those others she meets every day who are struggling with their own questions and pain.

RELIGION, SPIRITUALITY, AND THE END OF LIFE

Humanity has used spirituality and religion for millennia as guides in contemplating questions of the unknown and in navigating the search for purpose. This becomes imminently real for individuals facing serious illness. An overwhelming majority of patients with advanced cancer say that their religion and spirituality help them cope with their illness.[5] The use of religion as a coping mechanism can provide comfort, control, meaning, and even personal growth during times of peril. This remains true even in the current culture with the rising proportion of Americans who claim to be "spiritual but not religious" or even "none of the above."

Before we go further, we need to be sure what it is we are talking about. The term "spirituality" refers to the interior life, the search for personal identity and how one is related to others, to the cosmos, to the transcendent, to the divine. "Religion" defines, categorizes, and codifies that search and that life, using sacred texts, stories, teachings, and rituals. Put succinctly, spirituality is about questions and journey; religion is about answers and destination. In their spiritual quest, many people value the structure and guidance provided by religion, seeing these as helpful, even vital, in their spiritual understanding. Others, because of individual philosophy, or perhaps from negative experiences with religious persons or institutions, find the rules and boundaries of religion irrelevant or even oppressive. As each individual's life is singular, each person's inner self and search is unique.

When death approaches, these inner questions and struggles acquire greater urgency, but the time available for exploration and contemplation shortens. At this critical juncture, just when inner assurance is most desired, long-suppressed voices of distress may clamor to be heard, and long-utilized defense mechanisms may become insufficient for the existential assaults. The uncovering of long-hidden uncertainties can be the initial step toward answers and healing, but it can also produce spiritual torment. Inner spiritual and religious needs of the dying often become major or even primary sources of suffering. The US government recognized this when it established spiritual care as one of the five essential services each hospice must provide.

This interior, spiritual life is the part of us that seeks answers and meaning, that yearns for the "peace" in "peaceful death." As this inner part of our being is uniquely personal, it is difficult to quantify or measure. Accordingly, most research into the relationships between spirituality and dying have limited their questions to those of religion. Religiosity is easier to measure than a more nebulous term like "spirituality." As we will see below, these studies have produced valuable information and insight, but we are only beginning to understand this complex and essentially human dynamic.

Reliance on religion as a coping strategy strongly informs decisions made during illness and at the end of life. One fascinating study of healthy people provides insight into how Americans think about these issues. Those interviewed were told to imagine that they had suffered a life-threatening injury and then were asked about how religion would influence the choices they made. Most said that their religious beliefs would guide their medical decisions. Significantly, more than half held that God could heal them even if the doctors said that further medical efforts would be futile.[6] These data show that personal faith provides comfort and assurance for people who are seriously ill as well as guidance and even fantastic hope for those facing mortality. But do religion and spirituality actually affect the way people die, and if so, how?

Researchers use the term "positive religious coping" to designate the beneficial use of faith in dealing with illness and death. This can be expressed in many ways; one example would be someone who says, "I rely on God's love and care to get me through times of crisis." As suggested above, positive religious coping is a commonly employed and successful method of inner defense against impending danger and is usually viewed as a healthy form of psychological adaptation.

I began hospice work with a preconception that the patients who were more religious would have more peaceful deaths, would "know where they were going," and would be more likely to accept their mortality, less likely to scratch and claw for every extra hour of life. But that is not the case. Sure, stereotypic elderly persons, reading their Bible, comfortably accepting and even welcoming death do exist, exemplifying what many of us would hope our dying would be like, but I don't encounter them very often. In my clinical experience, there is little correlation between religiosity and peaceful death. This contradiction between my expectations and observations has been witnessed and studied by many others, who have shown, for example, that those whose religious faith is deeply held are less likely to execute advance directives or make decisions to limit care and are more likely to receive aggressive medical interventions near death, just the opposite of my preconceptions.

The patterns and magnitude of the relationships between positive religious coping and choices at the end of life was the subject of a recent large study. Patients with advanced and worsening cancer, as well as their spouse or other caregiver, were interviewed about how they coped with their illness and impending end of life. The investigators then followed these patients and their caregivers for the remainder of their lives, which ended, on average, about four months from the first interview. After the death, review of the medical records and repeat interviews with the surviving caregivers revealed what decisions had been made, what care had been provided, and what the dying experience had been like.

The patients who reported a high level of positive religious coping were more likely to acknowledge that their disease was, indeed, terminal and that their spiritual needs were being supported. But this realistic recognition of prognosis and sense of sustainment seemed at a disconnect when compared with care decisions made by and for these patients. Those with the highest levels of positive religious coping received intensive care aimed at prolonging life, including being placed on a mechanical ventilator, three times as often as those with a lower reliance on religion. In the United States, highly religious people, knowing they are dying, choose and receive aggressive, often futile medical interventions overwhelmingly more often than those whose personal faith is less vital.[7]

In patients with advanced and terminal disease, like those in this study, the use of aggressive care at the end of life usually does not keep people alive longer, and it is hugely expensive. In addition, patients who receive these types of treatment have lower quality of life during their final days, as was illustrated back in chapter 1. Also, their surviving caregivers have a higher risk of complications and suffering in their bereavement. Because of these things, many health care experts and medical ethicists use words like "futile," "unhealthy," or even "dangerous" when describing this type of care for people at the end of life. For people to knowingly choose this approach, they must perceive positive benefits or perhaps hold alternative values or points of view that act as a counterweight to these strong negative effects.

Why Do Religious People Choose More Aggressive Care When Dying?

One possible factor influencing the choices religious people make in their medical care stems from the opinions and actions of their clergy. Whether and how this interaction occurs is the focus of ongoing research. A study conducted a few years ago offers an initial and intriguing glimpse, though it probably raises more questions than it answers. A randomly selected group of American clergy persons received a survey to assess their agreement with statements of "life-prolonging religious values," including belief in miracle cures, sanctity of life, trust in divine control, and redemptive suffering. They were also asked to recall the congregant who had most recently died, what medical decisions they had discussed with the patient, and where that parishioner spent the last week of life. The 1,005 clergy who responded to the survey were overwhelmingly Christian and largely from various Protestant denominations. The majority affirmed the possibility of God performing a miracle despite a terminal diagnosis (86%) and the importance of continuing medical treatment because of the sanctity of life (54%). Those clergy with strong endorsement of these values had fewer end-of-life conversations with terminally ill congregants and had discussed entering hospice only half as often as the other clerics surveyed. [8]

Another insight came from a study of patients with serious chronic medical conditions (colorectal cancer, diabetes, congestive heart failure), who were asked about their end-of-life preferences, completion of advance directives, religious affiliation, importance of religion, beliefs about who or what determines length of life, and other values. [9] This report showed a distinction based on the concept of who or what controls issues of human life and death. Those who stated that God controls when death will occur were much less likely to engage in advance care planning or even to have informal discussions with relatives about their preferences. Conversely, adherence to the idea that death is an inevitable, but natural, part of life increased the likelihood of naming a surrogate, such as a DPAH, to speak for them if they are incapacitated and executing advance directives to be sure that death occurs when nature intends.

The idea that individual destiny, especially as it regards issues of living and dying, is controlled or at least strongly influenced by forces exterior to ourselves is pervasive in religious thought. The ancient Greek idea of fate and the Eastern religious concept of karma are two familiar examples. The Western monotheistic traditions offer much support for this idea. In the Hebrew scriptures, Job acknowledges that mortals' "days are determined, and the number of their months is known to [God]."[10] And the Koran says, "No one can die before his appointed term except in accordance with the law of God."[11]

Closely tied to the idea of God being in control of longevity is the issue of what happens to a person after their body is no longer alive. The question of the existence of an immortal soul, spirit, or anima, apart from the physical body and brain, is far beyond our scope here, but the idea of such is pervasive in most religious traditions and in much popular culture. What happens to that soul (the word I will use as it is the one most commonly applied in the American vernacular) after the death of the physical body has been hypothesized by every culture since antiquity.

Sometimes the afterlife is described as an empty state: the writer of the biblical book of Ecclesiastes says that "the living know that they will die, but the dead know nothing."[12] More often, though, religious teachings on afterlife include some type of judgment, of reward or punishment related to the actions, behavior, or belief of the dying person. Norse mythology described Valkyries who chose who would die in battle and carried selected slain warriors to Valhalla. *The Tibetan Book of the Dead*, described in more detail in chapter 7, describes a complex and perilous landscape that the departed one must successfully traverse in the search for the womb by which one will be reborn.[13] The auspiciousness of that womb, the character of one's new life, is dependent on one's karma, the result of actions during previous lives as well as the state of mind at the time of dying. Most Americans are familiar with the idea of a judgment based on one's actions during life, whether they acknowledge that future life as a reality or not. The most ordinary form of this conception is that of a binary afterlife, often called Heaven and Hell, in which those who meet the divine requirements are accepted and celebrated, while those who do not are disowned and tortured forever. The doctrines of religions define the criteria that will be used in judgment and therefore the actions individuals should take during life so as to receive the reward and not the punishment. Jesus illustrated it this way:

> There was a rich man who was dressed in purple and fine linen and who feasted sumptuously every day. And at his gate lay a poor man named Lazarus, covered with sores, who longed to satisfy his hunger with what fell from the rich man's table; even the dogs would come and lick his sores. The poor man died and was carried away by the Angels to be with Abraham. The rich man also died and was buried. In Hades, where he was being tormented, he looked up and saw Abraham far away with Lazarus by his side. He called out, "Father Abraham, have mercy on me, and send Lazarus to dip the tip of his finger in water and cool my tongue; for I am in agony in these flames." But Abraham said, "Child, remember that during your lifetime you received your good things, and Lazarus in like manner evil things; but now he is comforted here, and you are in agony."[14]

What about Suffering?

The belief in a God who is in control and who judges individuals according to belief or performance, then, leads to a third issue addressed by religious teaching: that of the meaning of suffering endured during the last phase of life. Religious texts and teachers struggle, as do all schools of thought, to identify the sources of pain and suffering and to clarify what meaning, if any, they hold. The idea that intense pain, angst, or existential distress might be meaningless is abhorrent to traditions that see order and purpose in reality. The deep philosophical questions surrounding human suffering are far beyond our purposes; a few examples will have to suffice. Buddhism, which sees all of physical life as suffering, teaches that everything has a cause, so what one is experiencing now is the result of previous events and actions done by or to us; it is our karma. In the monotheistic traditions, suffering is sometimes seen as caused by God but more often as the result of a world system in rebellion against the divine will.

For the individual who is suffering, the question is not one of philosophy or theology but of personal threat. One pervasive perspective, going back to prehistory, is that suffering is punishment for inferior performance. If one is experiencing severe pain or distress, it must indicate defective morality or lack of trust, because obviously the innocent faithful one would be spared these afflictions. Many patients ask, "What did I do to deserve this?" This question was posed most intensely by Jesus, as he was undergoing crucifixion, when he called out, "My God, my God, why have you forsaken me?"[15]

The example of Jesus and of the myriad others who, despite their innocence, have endured torture and execution should squelch any adherence to the concept that suffering is a cosmic judgment. Yet that exact idea remains prevalent, especially among those who are religious. It is hard to escape; it appeals to the human hope that the universe must somehow be a place of justice, that it makes sense. We buy it because we all carry secrets; we all have closet skeletons. We share a sense of guilt as well as a fear that at some point we will pay because of that guilt. The Torah warns, "Be sure your sin will find you out."[16] For someone whose death is approaching rapidly, there is precious little time to atone for transgressions, relieve guilt, and avoid punishment. The patient may make promises like a soldier in a foxhole. They may vow to change their beliefs and behavior, hoping, like the pagan who sacrifices a goat, to propitiate the deity with the power to punish.

Another common teaching is that suffering serves as a purgative, a burning away of evil tendencies, to produce, in the suffering one, a divinely acceptable purity. Thankfully, public self-flagellation is uncommon these days, but the idea behind it persists. In the survey of clergy alluded to above, many endorsed the idea that enduring painful medical treatment was of value because of the redemptive nature of suffering.[17] Occasionally I have encountered patients who delayed or avoided taking painkillers, believing that experiencing and accepting their pain was what God expected of them. The writer of the New Testament Letter of James advised those who faced suffering to "consider it nothing but joy,"[18] as enduring difficulties helps produce a mature and complete follower of God.

Another religious approach to the meaning of suffering is to ignore issues of punishment or purging, to simply accept what occurs as part of a mysterious divine or cosmic evolution. This view sees suffering as simply part of the present situation, an unavoidable characteristic of the human condition. These individuals usually accept and are grateful for whatever relief is offered and hope for the strength to endure, even grow from their pain.

Two Hypothetical Extremes

The religious conceptions discussed above, of a God who controls how long we live, who judges us, deciding on our eternal reward or torment, and who is somehow involved in the pain and suffering we endure, are prominent in the American psyche. How might these beliefs result in the desire for treatments like resuscitation and mechanical ventilation, even when they are futile and cause more pain? And, perhaps more important for the individual believers, do these beliefs assuage the fears described earlier in this chapter? I offer two hypothetical extremes as illustrations.

If God is benevolent, a loving parent who accepts me despite my failings, I can feel assured that the choices God makes for me are trustworthy and will be the best for me. God's will, even if it includes severe suffering, will work for my good, and any pain I endure now will be compensated for with exceeding joy after I die. I don't want to limit the time I have to receive more of the blessings that God has in store for me. And, who knows? Maybe that blessing will be a miraculous cure; my staying alive might help bring that miracle about!

On the other hand, God may be judgmental, one who knows every dreadful thing that I have done, including those I've not told anyone. If I suffer, it is either as punishment for what I have done or else it is a test to see if I can measure up. Hopefully I'll do well enough dealing with this trial to eventually squeak by and avoid eternal damnation. If I doubt or question the dogmas I've been taught, that's another point against me, so I can't even think of going there. I need more time to show God how good I really am! And maybe, after I've suffered enough, God will cure me and give me another chance to do better.

In my work with the dying, I have seen examples of both extremes, as well as various admixtures of them, influencing how religious people approach the end of their lives. Thinking about choices for the end of life through the lenses of these extremes does clarify a bit why those who primarily use this kind of religion as a coping strategy do not tend to limit care and do tend to desire every opportunity for life extension, no matter what their view of the character of God.

But what about fear? We identified this as the primary emotion we hope will be dealt with by our spirituality. With each recited *Ave Maria*, fifty repetitions with each rosary, faithful Catholics plead, "Holy Mary, Mother of God, pray for us sinners, now and at the hour of our death." For many religious people, the ability to trust God for the best outcome can relieve them of the need to struggle with difficult decisions or to dread what is to come. But, as illustrated above, this is not always the case, and such an approach may increase pain and suffering. The major source of that suffering is what we identified above, acknowledgment of personal guilt and fear of not being acceptable to God. In other words, that which should bring comfort can increase distress.

As a hospice physician, I saw relief of suffering as my prime mission, and I felt frustrated when I saw patients and families enduring emotional and spiritual anguish, particularly when that suffering was caused or accentuated by religious guilt. Hospice chaplains report that those whose faith is rooted in dogma and correct belief and action, who are "religious but not too spiritual," suffer the most in the dying process.

No one should infer any antireligion sentiment in anything I have said here. I wrote above that many find religious traditions to be sources of profound comfort and meaning. I know this to be true because it has been so for many friends, relatives, and patients, and also because it is true for me. The essential point is whether one's religion is primarily a matter of intellectual assent to doctrines and beliefs or whether the essence of a person's faith has become understood and embodied (incarnated) in their being. It is often the time of peril, what St. John of the Cross called the "dark night of the soul," that both tests the validity of one's faith and initiates that essential process of incarnation.

MAGDALENA AND HEALING

Magdalena seemed relieved when she was admitted to the inpatient hospice unit. She came to our care after a long and difficult hospitalization for complications of her advanced ovarian cancer. The rampages of the disease and the effects of the chemotherapy had produced profound debilitation. The cancer had spread extensively throughout her abdomen, which was filled with fluid that had become impossible to drain. She joked about being "eighty-one years old and eight months pregnant!" Finally, her doctors had told her that there was no more they could do, and that she would die, likely within several weeks.

She said she was reassured because now she could relax. She was the matriarch of a large, devoted family and looked forward to living with her daughter and "putting my feet up and letting somebody else do the work for a change." The weight of the abdominal fluid combined with her weakened state made it difficult for her to get around, but we had no doubt that, with a little help from a home hospice team, her family could manage her care. She had pain from the abdominal distention and her long-standing arthritis, but this was easily controlled with simple medications. She couldn't eat much at a time and said that the cooks at our facility clearly needed to learn a thing or two, but she did enjoy the cannoli made from her own recipe that her daughter brought in (as did we!).

We couldn't figure out why things suddenly changed, why the relief was replaced by reticence about going home with her daughter. It had been a normal day; I made a minor adjustment of her pain medicines, the social worker discussed what equipment would be needed at home, and a Eucharistic minister from the local parish visited and provided communion. But Magdalena seemed distressed. Her daughter thought she was afraid of something and called her home parish priest to visit. What had been minor nuisance symptoms now became Magdalena's sole focus, reasons why she wasn't ready to leave the inpatient setting. We reassured her that by discharging her we were not abandoning her; the local hospice team would meet her at her daughter's home the same day she arrived, and they would be sure that she was safe, cared for, and comfortable. Reluctantly, Magdalena resigned herself to leaving in the morning.

But when I made early rounds the next day, she asked me if there was someone else that she could talk with about something that was bothering her. Fortunately, one of the hospice spiritual care coordinators, a Protestant minister, was visiting someone else in the unit and agreed to stop in. About a half hour later, he came back out of her room, smiling but with streaks of recent tears. Magdalena had revealed her secret; she had acknowledged and loved the aborted child from six decades earlier, had accepted the love and forgiveness her God had always been offering, and had allowed the wound to be opened so it could heal. Magdalena's fear of damnation was replaced by assurance of grace; now she could live, and now she could die.

ADDRESSING THE REAL QUESTION

Life coach Samir Selmanovic observed that "when we can't fit our life experience into our religion, something has to give, and life can't give."[19] Magdalena, as well as all the other Magdalenas I have known, showed me the intense pain that dogmatic religion can cause as well as the profound healing that can occur from it or in spite of it. The healing stems from openness to the depths of meaning and love that are the goal of the spiritual quest, the quest on which religion is but one guide. Many find peace within the faith they have held through their lives. If religions did not provide a basis for solace, a balm for pain, they would not have endured. Others, like Magdalena, must risk stepping outside the boundaries of their personal religious heritage and understanding to discover the yearned-for peace.

In treating physical symptoms, many hospices and hospice doctors use standing orders, algorithms, and cookbook-type approaches. These are tried-and-true solutions to common problems, answers to FAQs. The problem is, sometimes the patient, the symptom, doesn't read the cookbook. Sometimes the true problem is masked. In that case the treatment cannot work because it is aimed at something that is not the real issue. I'm sure Magdalena knew many profound truths, many answers from her Roman Catholic heritage; the problem was that the answers she knew did not address the questions she was asking, the fears she was experiencing. For a patient whose life is on the line, their questions, their fears, are the true need. If compassionate and well-meaning clergy provide pat advice or rote doctrines, like those Emily heard at Charlene's funeral, they may well not address the patient's need. What occurs too often then is that the patient thinks that their question is wrong, that their fear is irrational, heretical, or even worse, unimportant. This is one reason I grieve when a patient says they "don't need" to talk with the hospice chaplain. Cancer patients who report that they receive high levels of spiritual support from their own faith community are less likely to receive hospice care and more likely to undergo aggressive interventions and die in an intensive care unit than those receiving spiritual support from their medical team. Hospice spiritual care is the resource with enough spiritual and religious depth and understanding to totally focus on the needs of the patient and family without the need to defend a faith or doctrine. Rather than replacing or competing with a patient's clergy or other spiritual advisors, hospice chaplains bring expertise about the particular concerns of the dying to supplement and add perspective to the rich content of all faith traditions.

We started this chapter talking about fear. What the spiritual quest offers is the antithesis of fear: hope. The meaning of hope has been cheapened to the level of superficial wishes and fantasies. A child wishes for a pony as a birthday gift just as an adult wishes for a job promotion. We fantasize about an unexpected romance or winning the lottery. But hope is something deeper. Back in chapter 4 we saw that suffering is caused by a threat to the integrity of our personhood. Our defensive response to that threat is fear, the recognition that our strength, our abilities, are inadequate in the face of the impending disaster. Fear is the product of brokenness. Hope, on the other hand, is the assurance that, whatever occurs, we will be intact, we will be okay. My favorite definition of hope comes from radio interviewer and author Krista Tippett, who says it is "broken-hearted on the way to becoming wholehearted."[20] Against well-grounded hope, the Gobble-uns stand no chance.

7

WHAT DOES IT FEEL LIKE TO DIE?

Death is horrible and stupid and it can't be and it is.
— Richard Beard, *Lazarus Is Dead*

My father died twice; we buried him after the second time. The first time, Dad was doing one of the things that gave his life meaning: he was delivering a pickup load of food for the needy. When he stopped for too long at an intersection, the driver behind tooted politely, then laid on the horn, and finally got out of the car to investigate. Dad's body had slumped over and was wedged between the steering wheel and the door. The irritated driver–turned–good Samaritan pulled Dad from the cab to the roadbed, established that he was unresponsive and pulseless, called 911, and started CPR. Some minutes later the squad arrived, initiated advanced cardiac life support, reestablished a pulse, and rushed him to the local hospital emergency room, where he was stabilized and promptly transported to a regional medical center.

It was several hours before I had a chance to see him. Mom had taken the first few minutes allowed to visitors; she told me Dad was not awake and was on a breathing machine. Nobody knew just how long he had been without effective circulation, how long his brain had been starved of oxygen, and whether he would ever wake up. My first look at this previously strong, vibrant man lying limply unaware of his surroundings was enough of a shock to put me into my coping strategy of "doctor mode." He showed no reaction when I pinched his nail beds as hard as I could; was this the first time I had physically hurt my father? Even more worrisome to me was the absence of what are called primitive reflexes, like the one that makes you blink when something touches your eyeball. It takes about three days after a cardiac arrest before it is possible to accurately predict the severity of brain injury, but looking at my dad then, I could not imagine or even hope he would return to being his former self. I remember telling my youngest sister on the phone that the man we both knew as our father was not coming back.

My oldest sister took a different approach. Her career had been in hospital nursing, so she understood what I was worried about. But she said, "I can't wait until Dad wakes up, so he can tell us what he saw, what happened while he was dead." I was startled by this comment but then realized that she, too, had found a safe place in which to process what was happening; for her it was the world of the mystical and the miraculous. Eventually, our father did wake up. His heart was a bit the worse for wear, though it managed to keep him going for another eight years; even more surprising, his brain seemed totally intact. He remembered nothing about his heart attack or of any visions or experiences. But he became a different person; we all noticed it. Dad believed he had received a miraculous granting of further life, and his faith told him that this meant there were changes to be made, there was life to be lived, all in gratitude for that divine gift. I've never been sure if the changes I saw in my dad were because of this conscious repentance or maybe because something did happen, something too distant, awful, or wonderful to be remembered.

IMAGES OF AFTERLIFE

Whether there is life beyond bodily death is a current and an ancient question. Socrates, as he was concluding his defense, said that "death is one of two things. Either it is annihilation, and the dead have no consciousness of anything; or, as we are told, it is really a change: a migration of the soul from this place to another."[1] Philosophical and religious traditions have hypothesized, studied, and developed dogmas on life after death, but we really are left with just these same two options: either death is a finality, as we assume it is for a squashed beetle or an uprooted and discarded house plant, or else it is a transformation, a transition to another state of being.

Commonly cited evidence about the possibility of conscious existence after physical death comes from those who report "near-death experiences," the kind of message my sister was hoping to hear from my dad. Accounts of adventures beyond the grave date back to ancient Greece; the earliest account is in Plato's *Republic*, from a time not much later than the death of Socrates. A man named Er, apparently killed in battle, roused himself from the funeral pyre and reported what he had seen as he was on a journey with many others. He had arrived at a place of judgment with two passageways in the earth. Individuals were coming and going in both directions, inquiring about conditions in the other world.[2] In the 2,500 years since Plato, a rich lore of stories relating metaphysical awareness among dying patients, their families, and those who care for them has accumulated. There are a multitude of testimonies of "near-death," "out-of-body," or simply eerie experiences that purport to provide a glimpse into another realm. Many of these contain rich imagery or symbolism, with personal detail, and make compelling reading. They have engendered a vocabulary I heard repeatedly at the bedside, the most common being telling the dying one to "go to the light." My science-based, rational mind is not certain what to make of these accounts. Are they miraculous reports from beyond the grave? Are they hallucinations? Or maybe they come from brain tissue starved of oxygen or side effects of drugs. For those who experience them, though, they are genuine, true, and important, and frequently cited as the reason for change in personal philosophy or behavior. Whatever they do or do not reveal about a possible metaphysical realm, they are the reported experience of the dying person and must be taken seriously. My practice was, as much as possible, to listen to the reports, share in the emotion and the meaning, and discern what these stories told me about my patient and also about my own ideas and insights. In the words of a lecturer I once heard, "Dying is not a problem to be solved; it is a mystery to be experienced."

In chapter 6, we encountered the religious idea of life after or beyond physical death. Archeological and anthropological studies of ancient cultures demonstrate the ubiquity of ideas of afterlife. Particularly familiar to Americans are the gods of the underworld in the Greek, Roman, Egyptian, and Hindu pantheons: Hades, Pluto, Osiris, and Yama, respectively. In the most ancient of the sacred texts of Western monotheism, the Hebrew book of Job, the place of the dead (Sheol), is described as a "land of gloom and chaos, where light is like darkness."[3] Christian and Muslim scriptures portray an afterlife in which the deceased are judged and then assigned to a place of either eternal comfort or everlasting agony. The Koran describes the reward for observant believers as "gardens under which rivers flow, and where, when they eat the fruits that grow . . . And they shall have fair spouses there, and live there abidingly."[4] The concept of a paradise to come is ingrained in our cultural psyche and was perhaps most poignantly described by Helen Keller when she said, "Dying is no more than passing from one room to another. But there's a difference for me, you know. Because in that room I shall be able to see." The images of endless punishment are equally vivid; the Koran depicts "a fire which will envelop them in its tent. If they ask for water they will be helped to liquid like molten brass that would scald their mouths."[5]

These familiar images of the "Heaven and Hell," binary afterlife suggest a state that is entered soon after the cessation of earthly life and that persists unchangingly forever. The Roman Catholic doctrine of Purgatory presupposes a third possibility, a temporary intermediate state between the two extremes, but this is just a transition phase to permanent bliss. A much more active and transitional afterlife is envisioned in many Eastern religions, whose thanatology is often referred to as reincarnation. One such tradition is that described in intricate detail in *The Tibetan Book of the Dead*.[6] In this ancient text, the odyssey of the dying one begins before the moment of physical death and continues through the bardo, the state of expedition between death and rebirth. En route, the departed encounters benevolent and wrathful deities, opportunities and obstructions to the successful completion of the journey to a propitious womb for entry into the next physical life. The text is directed to the counselor or guru at the bedside, providing signs and timelines indicating what the dying one is encountering on the journey as well as instructions and advice the guru should speak to the departed at each stage along the way.

Mark Twain, even as he disavowed belief in immortality, foresaw death as a transition to nothingness, the same nothingness that was his "existence" before his birth. He looked forward to this ending of being with as much optimism as many religious anticipate paradise:

> Annihilation has no terrors for me, because I have already tried it before I was born—a hundred million years—and I have suffered more in an hour, in this life, than I remember to have suffered in the whole hundred million years put together. There was a peace, a serenity, an absence of all sense of responsibility, an absence of worry, an absence of care, grief, perplexity; and the presence of a deep content and unbroken satisfaction in that hundred million years of holiday which I look back upon with a tender longing and with a grateful desire to resume, when the opportunity comes.[7]

Visioning, Hallucinations, Agitation

A guru using *The Tibetan Book of the Dead* to guide his charge through the stages of death has information on what the departing one is encountering and how to provide advice and assistance. Otherwise, the experience of dying, especially after most consciousness has departed, is a mystery to those observing the process. Many a family member, watching their dying loved one, has pondered, "I wonder what she is going through." What do I, as the physician, do when my patient, or their family, reports sights, sounds, smells, or other sensations that are not part of physical reality as we know it? When the unresponsive patient reaches their arms out, are they greeting a long-lost loved one, fending off a frightening demon, or simply stretching uncomfortable muscles?

We hospice professionals are admittedly inconsistent in the interpretation and advice we provide to families. When a dying patient appears to be looking beyond the others present in the room, reaching out to something or someone the others do not see, and seems to be comforted or happy, we call it "visioning." Visioning is usually managed with reassurance to the family and even celebration that the patient seems to be in a better place. But if the same patient seems afraid, fighting caregivers, screaming out, we term it "terminal restlessness" or "agitation" and treat it with powerful medicines to make it stop. I suspect that much visioning and agitation are two parts of the same spectrum, similar phenomena, even though we approach them differently. Maybe they are encounters with a metaphysical existence, maybe they are hallucinations, maybe they are effects of disease or drugs. Since we must admit that we really don't know what is happening, what is being experienced, the best we can offer is to evaluate whether the patient appears to be suffering, and if so, to try to alleviate it, and if not, to just observe or even celebrate what is happening.

THE MOMENT OF DEATH

As discussed in the introduction of this book, each person has an idea, detailed or poorly formed, of what they think, hope, or believe happens when our bodies die. That idea, that expectation, informs how one thinks about the time of death. Depending on this vision, the time of dying might be welcomed, dreaded, or ignored. Having been witness to the passing of multiple individuals, I continue to find that moment poignant, mysterious, even sacred.

From the medical and legal standpoints, death occurs at a specific time: the moment that the heart stops and breathing ceases (or in some cases the time when the death of the brain was declared). On each death certificate I complete, I enter a specific time of death. Before that minute, the patient is a person, with all rights and privileges inherent thereto. After that minute, it is a corpse. But, of course, that is not the whole truth. The person is loved by those next to the bed just as much after death as before. Frequently, before the moment of passing, family members talk among themselves; immediately afterward they speak to the body, often with caresses and expressions of love. Somehow, the person who has died remains.

Our secular and religious practices conform to this idea. In some Buddhist traditions, the body is allowed to remain in place, or as undisturbed as possible, for a period of hours to allow for the uninterrupted gradual exit of the person from the corpse, often with a window open for uninhibited egress. For many American funerals, the body is dressed up in its best clothing, surrounded with flowers, displayed, visited, and touched as a sacred object. When memorial services are held, whether shortly or more distantly after the death, the corpse, ashes, or at least a photograph is present, not just as a reminder that such a person lived but also as a demonstration that this individual is somehow still present and cared about.

The moment of dying, though, is engrained in our ideas and culture. We've all seen countless scenes on television and in movies, images of people who are alive and uttering profound last words one second, slumped over and gone the next. We seem to acknowledge both the tangibility of a specific instant of death and a real presence of that person that persists after bodily life has ceased. But what does the one who dies experience during that time of departure?

We alluded to the reports of near-death experiences earlier in this chapter as a possible source of evidence of what the dying person goes through, but, of course, the people making those reports did not complete the process; they did not die. Artistic representations of dying may depict angelic beings escorting the deceased one upward, or perhaps a wraith-like caricature of the dead body emerging from the corpse. My oldest sister, the one who wanted to hear Dad's report from the other side, quoted scripture to describe what she thought dying was like; in the Gospel according to John, Jesus says, "I will come again and will take you to myself, so that where I am, there you may be also."[8] The image of being transitioned in an instant into the realm and presence of the divine is widely held and undoubtedly reassuring.

Another comforting metaphor describing what happens at physical demise is that of rest. Even those not familiar with the Latin phrase *requiescat in pace* use its modern English versions, "rest in peace" or even "RIP," as shorthand for the fact of death and the wish that the departed one is not bothered by the tribulations of physical life. This image was beautifully expressed by John Milton in *Paradise Lost*:

> How gladly would I meet,
> Mortality my sentence, and be earth
> Insensible, how glad would lay me down,
> As in my mother's lap? There I should rest,
> And sleep secure.[9]

Not all the descriptions of the dying transition are so encouraging. An older translation of *The Tibetan Book of the Dead* includes, in archaic but stark language, the moment the departing soul recognizes that death has come: "Thou seest thy relatives and connexions and speakest to them, but receivest no reply. Then, seeing them and thy family weeping, thou thinkest, 'I am dead! What shall I do?' and feelest great misery, just like a fish cast out [of water] on red-hot embers. Such misery thou wilt be experiencing at present. But feeling miserable will avail thee nothing now."[10]

The idea of suffering like a fish suffocating and burning on a charcoal grill is terrifying, and if that is what dying is like, we do well to fear it.

So, is the moment of dying an exalting transportation into a divine metaphysical realm, an agonizingly terrifying realization of hopelessness, the beginning of a well-deserved rest, or just an extinction? We must admit that we don't know. To close this section, then, I have chosen to share two of my favorite descriptions of death. The Chinese philosopher Lao Tzu reportedly said, "What the caterpillar calls the end, the world calls a butterfly." But perhaps the most honest statement about dying is attributed to Woody Allen, who is quoted as saying, "It's not that I'm afraid to die, I just don't want to be there when it happens."

FROM THE HEROIC TO THE EROTIC

Seared into every person's consciousness is respect, even devotion to an ideal of sacrificing one's own life because of or for some overarching cause. When the fallen are killed in the service of the nation to which we claim allegiance, our collective respect achieves a religious quality. Americans teach their children Lincoln's words at Gettysburg because they articulate exactly that point; they declare that the blood spilled on that battlefield acted as a fertilizer for a new imagining of the American republic. Taking a lead slug in the belly is transformed from an experience of horror to a sacred act.

For some who die in battle, that is exactly the point. They, either by plan or happenstance, find themselves with a choice of risking themselves for the benefit of comrades, cause, or country. They are awarded medals, recognition of outstanding heroism. But these are the great exception; most of the time the one who is killed has been trained to follow orders, to act despite the terror, the loathing of what one will do, what will occur. To these, did dying feel like a sacrificial act? The meaning of their deaths is ascribed by the survivors. If their side was victorious, their deaths were glorious; they died that others might live. But the Confederate casualties at Gettysburg were just as dead, had acted just as bravely and as patriotically as those Union soldiers whose cemetery Lincoln dedicated that day.

But honor, duty, and patriotism are not the only emotions that overwhelm, that affect how one's dying feels. From the story of Romeo and Juliet to the history of Bonnie and Clyde, the image of lovers dying together appeals to our romantic sensitivities. Even when lovers' deaths are not temporally close, we imagine the couple who shared love and life united somehow in an eternal embrace. We envision the one who has died previously as waiting, the moment of the partner's death as the beginning of the ultimate consummation of the relationship. Virtually every day the obituary column proclaims that some deceased couple is "together again."

All these images merge in the third act of Richard Wagner's opera *Tristan und Isolde*. Tristan, the paragon knight of Arthurian legend, was sworn to King Mark of Cornwall, who had married Tristan's love, Isolde. The machinations of the legends are too complex to review here, but at the climax of the story, Tristan lies in his own castle, fatally wounded, desperately hoping for Isolde to arrive, as she is gifted with healing powers. Isolde arrives to greet her beloved just as he breathes his last. She weeps over his corpse, remembering their night of passion, and demands of him to not die of his wounds but to awaken for just an hour, so they can be united again and die together in the act of love. But, instead, she slumps senseless over his body and is no more.

WHAT DOES IT FEEL LIKE TO BE DYING?

Since the only experts on what it is like to die are those who have accomplished it, everything presented thus far is, by definition, hypothetical. But by being with, observing, and listening to those who are reaching the end of their lives, we can discover a sense of what it might be like to be a dying person. This is not true on a scientifically accurate level, if there is such a thing in the realm of this intensely individual experience, but on an experiential and emotional plane. Since it is fear—of the unknown, of suffering, or of unearthing the deep parts of ourselves—that largely prevents us from facing our mortality, the domains of experience and emotion are the appropriate fields for this exploration.

In order to encounter those areas in ourselves, it is necessary to do more than just sit and read words and sentences. The remainder of this chapter is a guided exercise adapted from one used in many hospices and end-of-life conferences as a way for participants to encounter the inner experience of dying. You will need about twenty minutes to do this, and it is more effective to do it without interruption, so if that isn't possible for you right now, skip ahead and come back to it when you can give it time and attention. I strongly recommend carrying out this exercise without reading it first. If you just read through it to get on to the next chapter, you'll probably understand a bit of its underlying design and purpose, but you won't encounter the emotional impact. If you don't do it, you won't get it!

This exercise is a worksheet; a form is available online,[11] but if you prefer, use any sheet of paper on which you will list fifteen items in five categories of three items each. First, write down three of your favorite material possessions, stuff you have that you like. Next enter three activities you enjoy participating in, things you like to do. Don't spend too much time trying to get the correct items on the list. There are no "right" answers; the first things that pop into your head are just fine. Now enumerate three favorite body parts. The best question ever posed to me by an audience member was when someone asked, "Do they have to be on your own body?" Your answers are your own, so, whatever! Following this, list three values you hold as important. And, to complete the worksheet, record the names of three people whom you love. Once your overall list of fifteen items is complete, you're ready to proceed.

You are reading this, so you have not died, but you have experienced losses of various sorts—everyone has. Everyone who dies loses everything. It doesn't matter if the death is sudden or protracted, agonizing or peaceful; when we die, we leave everything and everyone behind. How does it feel to lose that which is precious? What might it be like to awaken each day and recognize that there is yet one more thing you can no longer call your own? What happens when your career, the ability to drive, movement without pain, sexual intimacy, being able to eat, continence, privacy, consciousness, are all taken from you?

✷ ✷ ✷

You think that maybe you've finally arrived! You are in your mid-fifties, happily married, your daughter just graduated from college. Your boss has told you that your application for promotion is likely to be approved. You have always been careful with your finances, so, except for a few years left on your mortgage, there is little debt. Maybe you can try to relax a little now, do some of the things you always told yourself you'd do when your schedule was less demanding. Yes, it's time to celebrate life instead of always working at it. You and your spouse take a few days in the high desert of New Mexico, where you spent your honeymoon; the two of you have always loved the landscapes, the restaurants, and the art galleries.

You take a drive north out of Taos, up to the bridge over the gorge of the Rio Grande. You've found this stark and abrupt chasm mesmerizing in the past, and it lives up to your memory. The two of you walk along the edge, pausing occasionally for selfies or to take shots of each other in the bright New Mexico sunshine. What is it that your spouse is frowning about as you pose for her? "No, I don't think my eyes are yellow; it must just be the light." But when you look at the photo, well, maybe they are. "Yes, in this selfie of the two of us, my eyes are not as white as yours. They do look a little yellow." On your worksheet, cross off one of the fifteen items on your list.

On the drive back into town, the two of you talk about this, uncertain of its significance but knowing that it is not good. You have heard about people who had this, what do you call it, jaundice. As you eat dinner together, you can't relax enough to appreciate your steak, even with the assistance of a superb Cabernet. "Oops, maybe I shouldn't even be drinking this. Isn't jaundice a sign of a problem with my liver?" Your spouse says that your eyes don't look yellow now, so you try to relax and enjoy it. But as soon as you're back in your hotel room you are on the web trying to find out anything you can about jaundice. Should you go to the urgent care center you saw on your drive back? You feel as good as you ever have, so there can't be anything seriously wrong, can there? Cross off another item.

In the morning, you awake refreshed, surprised that you slept so well. You examine your eyes in the mirror as you brush your teeth and can't quite convince yourself they are normal, but then you never looked that closely before. After breakfast, when you know the office will be open, you call your internist to ask for advice. You've always liked her; office visits usually start with a minute of catching up on what is happening with your daughter, Georgia, or the doctor's Doberman, Bosco. The receptionist says to expect a call back before the end of the day. But an hour later your phone rings; it is your internist, telling you that this problem needs attention quickly. One option is to go to the local emergency room, but you are scheduled to fly back home this afternoon anyway, and you don't want to get stuck in a hospital this far away. You tell her that you feel great and have no pain anywhere, but this doesn't seem to reassure her. "Okay," she says. "Travel safely. I'll order some blood tests and an abdominal ultrasound for tomorrow morning, so don't eat anything after midnight tonight. I'll arrange to see you before the end of the day, when we'll have the results." This isn't the reassuring tone she usually takes with you, and it is a little frightening. This trip hasn't turned out to be the celebration you thought it would be. Cross one more item off your list.

You're back on the web now, paying more attention this time. The words you find there are disturbing: "hepatitis," "gallstones," "cirrhosis," "cancer." Somehow you manage to get through the day, following your spouse, automaton-like, through airport security, boarding, finding your car, getting into bed. The thoughts that keep you awake, that invade your fitful dreams, swing wildly between images of being the victim of tragedy or of a cruel prank. Cross another item off your list.

You are at the lab when it opens, get your blood drawn, then go to the radiology suite for your ultrasound, which isn't scheduled for another two hours. The morning news program on the mounted television is so vapid you wonder why people watch it. Then you notice how hungry you are and remember that you haven't even had any coffee. The ultrasound tech is friendly, but she looks younger than your daughter; can she really know what she is doing? She squirts warmed jelly on your skin and runs a probe over it, first lightly then with more force, repeatedly asking you to hold your breath while she gets specific pictures. This gives you something to do, at least, and takes your mind off your hunger and your worries.

When you check in at your doctor's office, the receptionist says that Bosco had won Best in Breed at a show last weekend, but in the exam room, your internist doesn't want to talk much about it. Instead, she asks a myriad of questions: how you have been feeling, what and where you have eaten in the past weeks, whether you have any pain in your stomach or your back, and whether you've had unprotected sex with anyone besides your spouse. She agrees that your eyes look yellow, and she explains to you that jaundice shows up better in sunlight and disappears in fluorescent light, so that is why it seemed to come and go. Your blood tests show no sign of hepatitis or liver damage, but the bilirubin level is high. This happened with your daughter when she was born; they put her under a light to make it go away. She says that in adults it doesn't work that way. Bilirubin is a breakdown product of blood cells that get cleared by your liver; in your case, the tube that drains the liver, the bile duct, is blocked. The ultrasound shows that the blockage is caused by a tumor in your pancreas. "Is it cancer?" She says she can't tell yet but that it most probably is. "So, what do we do next?" She explains the next steps, gives you some information sheets, orders a CAT scan for the next morning, and arranges for you to see a gastroenterologist in the afternoon.

You are glad your spouse came along for this appointment, as there is no way you can remember anything you are hearing. After that "cancer" word, your mind went blank. The scan and appointment are at the university hospital downtown; that in itself emphasizes that this is serious. Delete another item from your list.

Another morning without breakfast, and then when you arrive for your scan, they give you a quart or so of chalky sludge to drink. The technicians here seem more impersonal, and the entire process exudes a sense of technical efficiency. They dismiss you with, "Okay, you can get dressed now." You find your way to the cafeteria for some breakfast, but just as you take your first sip of coffee, your phone goes off. It is the gastroenterology nurse, who says that another patient canceled their appointment, so they can see you in twenty minutes. You argue that you are starving, but he says that it is probably best if you don't eat before the visit anyway. Your spouse hastily finishes her bagel and coffee while your stomach does somersaults of anxiety.

At least this doctor has some gray hair! Of course, before you see her, a wet-behind-the-ears "student doctor" talks with you, does a drawn-out examination, and tries to look competent. You notice the certificates on the wall attest to the gastroenterologist having received multiple teaching awards. You ask the student about it and are told, "Oh, yes, she's the best! I was lucky to get this rotation with her!" You try a few more questions; your bilirubin level is 6.3 (normal is less than 1.2). The student says, "That's nothing; somebody yesterday had one of 27!" When the attending physician goes over the results with you, she seems both competent and caring. You feel like you're in good hands. You've been preparing for the worst, so this time you can listen to what she has to say. The tumor is almost certainly a cancer of the pancreas, though she says there are several types. The immediate problem is the bile duct blockage; she advises getting this taken care of today, especially since it is early and you have had nothing to eat. You are glad to start doing something other than just more tests. She explains that this will be part test, part treatment. She will go down your throat with an endoscope, take specialized ultrasound pic-

tures from the inside of your small intestine, obtain needle biopsies of the tumor, and open the bile duct, placing a stent to keep it
patent. You've got to wait until her clinic is over and she can get a
time slot in the endoscopy suite; that's fine with you because before the end of the day, you'll be on your road to getting better.

As you wander, looking for things to do around the hospital,
Georgia calls; she had a fender-bender accident this morning. She
is okay, just shaken up. You hand the phone to your spouse. You've
not let anybody else know what is going on, and you just can't
bring yourself to talk with her right now. Cross another entry from
your list.

You don't remember anything about the procedure except the
start of the IV and the words, "Let's start with sixty and two." In
the recovery room, your spouse is there, but now your stomach
hurts. The ginger ale and shortbread cookies taste like ambrosia.
After you are more awake, your doctor stops in and tells you that
she was able to do the biopsies and place the stent without difficulty. Your jaundice will clear in a few days. The bad news is that
the ultrasound showed that the tumor is invading the portal vein,
the large, vital vessel that drains blood from the intestine into the
liver, and this might prevent successful surgery. She says that the
best approach is for you to go to the GI oncology clinic where
there are several experts in this kind of cancer. Your brain is still a
bit fuzzy from the drugs, but the impact of what she is saying hits
you square in the face. This is bad. Cross off another item.

Was it just a week ago that you and your spouse were having
dinner at that great Mexican fusion place in Santa Fe, talking
about all the things you would do together, how you felt a sense of
freedom from financial and family frustrations you had been
through? This just came out of the blue, literally out of the high
sunny blue sky.

Isn't that just the way it is? Surprise occurrences can instantly
alter our ideas about the future. It might be an unanticipated raise
or a layoff, a touchdown or a career-ending knee injury, falling
madly in love or suffering a heart attack, buying a winning lottery
ticket or noticing that your eyes are yellow. Whatever ensues, it

will be different than we thought it would be. Life is changed, foreign, disorienting.

The GI oncology clinic meets on Friday; you are told to arrive at 9:00 and to expect to be there for most of the day. As you survey the waiting room, you seem to be the healthiest one there but also the most nervous. An oncology fellow spends about an hour with you, sorting through the story, doing another physical exam, collating all the test results, reviewing what will happen next, and outlining the questions that still need to be answered. You are happy when he tells you that your bilirubin level is now normal but are less thrilled with the news that the biopsy confirmed adenocarcinoma of the pancreas, the most lethal type of pancreatic cancer. The attending medical oncologist then comes in briefly and confirms what you just heard. You head back to the lobby, waiting to be called to see the surgeon and the radiation oncologist. This last one has multiple tattoos and a nose ring; you had thrown a fit when your daughter came home with a butterfly on her ankle!

It's now about 12:30. They tell you that they will all meet to discuss the findings in a tumor conference that afternoon, and if you can stay around until about 4:00 p.m., they can give you their recommendations. Or, if you'd prefer, you can go home, and they'll call you next week. There is no way you can imagine waiting through the weekend. You'll stay.

It is more like six o'clock when you get the call to go back to the clinic. The oncology fellow you started with confirms that the cancer involves the portal vein but that the surgeon thinks he might be able to remove it if the tumor shrinks with radiation and chemotherapy. He stresses how important this is, that successful surgical resection is your only hope for a cure. There are several variations on how the preoperative treatments could be given; he advises that you participate in a clinical trial comparing the combination of one of those standard regimens with an experimental drug. Everyone in the trial will take one capsule a day, but only half of the participants will get the active drug; the rest will get an inactive placebo. No, you can't pick which treatment you get; it is assigned by a computer in an office somewhere else. He gives you a twenty-page form to read with all the details of the study, including lists of possible side effects. You ask, "If I were your mother, what would you recommend that I do?" He is a bit flustered by this, but you like his answer, "Well, first of all I'm happy that my mom isn't facing this; you've already figured out this is a severe problem. But I do think that clinical trials offer the best hope for most patients with the added benefit of helping people in the future." People in the future—you picture the butterfly on Georgia's ankle as you sign the form. Take one more item off your list.

Treatment starts next week. You go for radiation planning in the meantime; this involves more scans, having a road map drawn on your skin and molds fashioned that will position you in the machine when you get your treatments. You find out that the tattooed radiation therapist isn't a freak; she has a delightful sense of humor, and all the staff clearly think she's the best there is. The morning your treatment is to start, a nurse places a long IV tube into your arm; she calls it a PICC line. You sit for hours in the chemotherapy suite; the chair is comfortable, the nurses seem nice, and the guy in the chair next to you gives you a thumbs-up when he introduces himself as Chester. He says he has colon cancer that has spread to his liver, and this is the third kind of chemotherapy they have given him for it. "I know you're nervous now, but just get in the routine and you'll be fine." You're thinking this is life and death, and he's talking about it as if it is nothing but a minor nuisance to get through. The nurses inject medicines to prevent nausea, then infuse one of the chemotherapy drugs over an hour or so. Next, they hook you up to a little pump that will be giving another chemotherapy drug continuously. They also give you a bottle of the experimental pills. They can't tell you whether this is the active drug or a placebo, and, in fact, nobody knows except that remote computer. You're just supposed to take one every day. Then you walk to the radiation suite; this time they place you in your mold in a machine that looks like something from Star Wars. Then the technician leaves the room and shuts a heavy door behind her. You can see her on a little TV screen; her voice comes through the speaker telling you the treatment will start now. The machine moves all around you, lights come on, the tech on the TV is sipping coffee, then it is over. This can't be right; it only lasted a couple minutes and you didn't feel a thing! Chester is right. The routine helps. He is there every week when you go in for your pump refill and one-hour chemotherapy infusion. You have radiation treatment every day, the techs get you in and out quickly, and you only need to wait there on the days you see the radiation oncologist. You are getting a little fatigued, your skin is getting dry, you've lost some weight and some hair, and you notice a bit of tingling in the tips of your fingers and toes, but overall this is nowhere near as bad as you thought it would be. You start to look forward to your chemotherapy days; everybody there is so upbeat! On the last day of treatment, you take candy in for the nurses and technicians.

Now it is time to recover and wait. The blood tests and repeat scans show that the cancer is probably smaller than before, and the surgeon tells you he thinks you should go ahead with the operation. You are happy about this but tell him you need more time to recover from the treatment you just finished. He advises against waiting. If you delay too long, there will be too much scarring from the radiation to do the surgery. But maybe what frightens you the most is that he tells you what he will do if it turns out that he can't remove the tumor. You've avoided that possibility. Chester's routine had worked so well for you that you had kept the big picture relegated to the background of your mind; the idea that your surgeon might need to retreat to "plan B" while he has your belly open reminds you of the stakes you are playing for. Cross one more thing off your list.

When you wake up in the recovery room after surgery, the first thing you notice is a pain like somebody stabbed you in the stomach, then it comes to you that your surgeon did exactly that. The staff there repeatedly look at the vital sign monitor above your head, remind you to take deep breaths, and tell you that the reason you feel like you need to pee is that you have a tube in your bladder. The cuff on your arm gets tight every couple of minutes. You vaguely recollect your surgeon talking with you but don't remember what he said. Then they wheel you to a hospital room; you notice your spouse walking beside the cart and appreciate the kiss planted on your forehead while you wait for the elevator. When you're finally settled in your hospital bed, your spouse is in the chair beside you. You figure out how to press the button on the machine that delivers a dose of pain medicine when you need it. Then you ask the big question. Your spouse takes a quick, startled breath. "Didn't the doctor tell you?" Then the tears flow. The cancer was too advanced to resect; there were even a few spots of cancer in your liver that must have been too tiny to see on the scan a couple weeks ago. So, it was plan B after all. He re-routed the bile ducts and intestine to be sure the jaundice didn't return and that list.

The medical oncology consult service comes to see you the day before your discharge. The fact of new spots in your liver is unwelcome news, but they offer to try some chemotherapy drugs that you had not received before. They say there is probably a one in four chance that this will help, though they stress that by "help" they mean make the cancer smaller or slow its growth, not cure it. For the first time, one of them mentions the "D" word, telling you that, though this treatment might help for a while, you will die from this disease. Cross another item off the list.

After you're up and around, you and your spouse take a walk in the woods to talk about the future. The treatment decision seems easy; a one in four chance of living longer is better than zero, certainly worth trying for. You'll take the chemotherapy, but then the arithmetic becomes clear: a one in four chance of treatment working means that there is a three in four chance that it won't. You clutch each other's hands even more tightly.

The sky is nearly as blue as it was that morning in New Mexico. As you walk together silently, there seems little that needs to be put into words. You have been so fortunate to have such a beautiful person share your life. You become aware of a gravelly voice in your mind and can't help humming along to a tune you hadn't thought of in years, with lyrics about green trees, red roses, and a wonderful world.

When you go to the GI oncology clinic the next week, the familiar suite seems changed somehow. You don't feel the same ambience of optimism. Maybe that was just in your head anyway. This new treatment will be given weekly and only take a couple hours. Sitting in your usual recliner, you try to sort out what else feels different. As you wheel your IV pole past the nurses' desk to get to the bathroom, you read the card on a bouquet of white roses on the counter; it is from Chester's widow. Cross one more entry off your list.

The first time I participated in an exercise like this, as I was getting down to just a few items left on my list, when told to cross them off I couldn't help but think, "Please, God, not that too!" After all, the items remaining are those most precious, most vital. And the thought of losing them, even in an imagined hypothetical situation, is threatening.

Is that what it is like to be dying? You may be trying to decide whether to cross off, say, your integrity or your daughter. You are sitting there doing this, suffering a little inside, and the rest of the world goes on. People around you watch TV, make dinner, argue, text their friends, all oblivious to what you are going through. The world goes on, not affected at all or even seeming to notice what is happening to you. Is that what it is like? Is that what it is like to die?

The treatment is going well, but you don't think it is working. Your appetite is still okay, but each week your weight is lower, until the week when it isn't. Then the subsequent week, it is a bit higher. The oncology fellow you first met, who has again rotated into the GI clinic, tells you that this is even worse news. The higher weight is because of fluid building up in your abdomen caused by the growth of the cancer in and around your liver. There is no reason to keep going with the chemotherapy, and the declining function of your liver prevents even considering any other treatment. He wants to call the palliative care team to see you, explaining that they are experts in the management of symptoms and in facilitating conversations about your goals and how to manage this last part of your life. This sounds like a good plan; you ask why it had not been mentioned before. He turns a bit flushed and stammers out an apology. "I guess we probably should have done that."

"So, Doc, how long have I got?" The fellow starts in on a technical explanation, mentioning all kinds of things that make it impossible to predict. But your spouse interrupts him. "That's all well and good, but it doesn't help. We really need to know what to hope for, what to plan on. Remember, at our first visit, when you were honest with us as you talked about your mom? We need that clarity now." His response shocks but really does not surprise you. "I'm sorry to say that we're talking in terms of weeks, not months." Cross another entry off.

You don't stay around to see the palliative care team; you just have to get out of that place. When you get home, you call your daughter but can't seem to get the words out. Your spouse takes the phone into another room to talk with her. By late evening, Georgia has made it there. You chide her that you are getting along fine so she didn't need to interrupt her life right now. "But this is my life, you guys. What else matters more right now?" Your mind comes up with parental advice about making sure she thinks about her future and what is best for her, but you swallow the words, feeling more loved by her than ever before. You must have done something right in raising her; how can you even imagine leaving her behind? Scratch off another item.

The next morning an intake nurse for a hospice agency calls. She says that after you left the clinic yesterday, the oncology fellow sent them a referral. She wonders if she can come to the house and talk. Your daughter is the one on the phone; you vigorously wave your hands to try to get her to head them off, but she covers the phone and says, "It can't hurt to listen" and makes an appointment for the afternoon.

You're not sure what you expected, but it wasn't this. The intake nurse seems to know exactly the questions to ask. At one point your spouse tears up and asks, "Why is it that nobody has ever asked us these things before?" She goes over what hospice has to offer, how it is paid for, what it will be like. You had thought of hospice as a place to go to die, but she is talking about making sure your life is as good as it can be. She doesn't sugarcoat anything but remains upbeat. Your spouse and daughter are sold on it; you're not so sure. "This sounds like a lot of effort and expense when I'm going to be dead in a few weeks anyway." Her response is perfect: "Then we'd better get started right away."

The next morning you are introduced to your hospice nurse, the social worker, two volunteers, a minister, and home health aides. With you and your family, they develop a plan for your care, instruct you on how to manage symptoms and situations, some of which you'd never thought of, and make sure you know how to access them at any time.

Friends and neighbors begin nearly incessant calls, visits, cards, even casseroles, but before long, that drops off. You find yourself paying more and more attention to those people and ideas that are most important to you, and you wonder what seemed so vital that took up so much of your time before. Your new perspective makes you think that maybe you are learning how to die. But the real irony is that you are also just now learning how to live.

But at night you are awakened by your fears and doubts. What was it all about anyway? Someone else will get the job promotion you were expecting. Someone else will walk your daughter down the aisle. You won't be there for your grandson's first home run or, more important, for all the times he strikes out. And worst of all is the deep unspoken fear: that you will be forgotten. Cross the last item off your list.

IVAN ILYCH AND YOU

In his novella *The Death of Ivan Ilych*, Leo Tolstoy introduces us to his protagonist, a midlife successful official who develops new symptoms, gets treated by the doctors of his day, deteriorates, and eventually dies. This short work can be read in one sitting, and, based on my experience with the dying, it is honest and accurate.

Ivan Ilych recognizes that as he is dying, he is doing it alone. "Those about him did not understand, or refused to understand, and believed that everything in the world was going on as usual. This thought tormented Ivan Ilych more than anything. He saw that his household, especially his wife and daughter who were absorbed in a perfect whirl of visiting, had no conception at all and were annoyed with him for being so depressed and exacting, as though he were to be blamed for that."[12]

His loneliness was worsened by those who avoided the truth, trying to protect him.

"Whether it was morning or evening, Friday or Sunday, made no difference, it was all one and the same: gnawing, agonizing pain never ceasing for an instant, the consciousness of life inexorably ebbing away but not yet gone; the relentless approach of that ever dreaded and hateful death, which was the only reality, and all this lying going on at the same time."[13]

As he found he could no longer count on his family or even his doctors for truth and solace, he also questioned the faith that had been essential to his life:

He wept at his own helplessness, at his terrible loneliness, at the cruelty of man, the cruelty of God, at the absence of God. "Why hast Thou done this? Why hast Thou brought me to this? Why, why dost Thou torture me so dreadfully?" He did not expect an answer, and yet wept because there was no answer and could be none.[14]

At his end, he found resolution, but not answers.

"What is this? Can it be true that it is death?" And the inner voice answered: "Yes, it is true."—"Why these agonies?" And the voice answered, "For no reason—they just are so." Beyond and besides this there was nothing.[15]

8

ENVISIONING YOUR OWN DEATH

Death, then, being the way and condition of life, we cannot love to live if we cannot bear to die.

—William Penn, 1693

I've envied Tom Sawyer because he got to watch his own funeral. The townspeople had given him and his friends Joe Harper and Huckleberry Finn up for dead, but they had only been off playing at being pirates for a few days. The community gathered to collectively mourn the loss of the three young lives. The boys, having spied out what was going on in the village during the time of their truancy, hid themselves in the unused gallery of the church and watched the proceedings before eventually revealing themselves as alive, well, and present. What they learned from this escapade was that they were missed, they were cared about, and they were loved. Even the essentially parentless Huck Finn realized that people cared about him. [1]

Tom had thought about dying before, mainly with the idea that, after his death, people would realize how much they cared about him and that they would be sorry for the mistakes they had made about him and the abuses they had heaped on him. This is a common way that people think about their own death, especially during adolescence, but it is antithetical to what I am advocating and advising. Seeing one's death only in selfish and revengeful images ("I'll show them") leads to further anger and alienation. These images unfortunately characterize the thought processes of many a teenager who commits suicide or shoots up a school. A part of the tragedy of these all too common events is that they are a waste of both life and death. What our contemplations on death have shown us is that life is precious and that the completing of it can be a process of healing and wholeness.

ALLAN

Allan shouldn't have gotten lung cancer. He never smoked, and he jogged regularly—even ran marathons. But he became my patient with a type of cancer that progressively infiltrated the tiny air sacs of his lungs, destroying their ability to get oxygen into his bloodstream. The chemotherapy drugs I treated him with didn't have any effect. As the cancer grew in the face of everything we were throwing at it, his endurance and ability to breathe deteriorated to the point that he had to use an oxygen tank just to walk from one room to the next. He knew he was dying. His diseased lungs could not continue to support his life for many more weeks. He did his advance care planning, had the tough talks with his wife and children, and prepared to die.

Allan was a motivated patient who meticulously adhered to my recommendations, even pushing himself beyond what might have been thought reasonable, in order to squeeze as much living into the time he had left. He had to give up his job as director of development at a midwestern university and was no longer able to volunteer his time and energy in community development. Allan had summed up the purpose of his life as "I do love to serve."

Just a few days before what I expected would be Allan's final appointment with me, the FDA approved compassionate use of a drug called gefitinib for patients with refractory lung cancer. Allan was game to try anything, and, since the reported side effects of this drug were minimal, there seemed little reason not to complete the required forms and write the prescription. Allan had done his dying work; this was a "no lose" proposition. He accepted my recommendation and enrolled with a local hospice agency but also obtained the medicine and made a follow-up appointment, though neither one of us expected that he would live to keep it.

ARS MORIENDI

If Americans talk about what they think dying should be like, one phrase that almost always emerges is that people should die "with dignity." If pushed to explain what that means, most talk about pain relief, being with family, and the other characteristics we've discovered throughout this book. For many, the essence of dignity is the maintenance of one's humanity, one's personhood, throughout the duration of life. A body of research, initiated by Canadian physician Harvey Chochinov, has explored just what dignity means and how it can be achieved by and for the dying. He and his colleagues have pioneered a unique and individualized psychotherapeutic intervention they term "dignity therapy."[2] The point of dignity therapy is to provide the dying one with an opportunity to reflect on things that matter most to them as well as those things they would most want others to think of when remembering them. One commonly used method is to create a legacy booklet or video in which a person can tell their story or stories.

The specifics of dignity therapy are novel, but the ideas at its core are ancient. The idea of the "good death" dates to antiquity; then as now, it centers on completing a life with integrity, of fulfilling one's true fate or calling. The Homeric hero who perished in battle was held in honor for his service, but more so because he had fulfilled his destiny. The Valkyries chose valiant fallen warriors and transported them to reward in Valhalla for the same reason. The Hebrew scriptures teach that the death of a faithful one is precious to God.[3] Common in all these is that the essence of human dignity is being true to one's self, the values one holds close, for as long as one lives.

In fifteenth-century Europe, the combined devastations of the Black Death and the Hundred Years' War raised, especially among clerics and their parishioners, the specter of divine judgment, a sense of God's displeasure and punishment. Along with this arose a more widespread awareness of the fragility of life. One's own demise, then, became a focus of concern; if death could come at any moment, it was important to prepare for it. One product of this age was an anonymous treatise titled *Ars Moriendi* (Art of Dying). The primary focus of this work was preparation for an afterlife, but it also indicated that following its instructions and advice would produce a peaceful ending of mortal existence. A revolutionary teaching in the *Ars Moriendi* was that the dying one needed to take an active role in anticipating death, to make the appropriate choices and take the necessary actions. One needed to focus on the approaching end of life and make the required active preparations. One's focus, then, on the coming end of life, with the resultant active preparations, defined the art of "dying well."

Thomas à Kempis, another fifteenth-century mystic, wrote, "Blessed is he that always hath the hour of death before his eyes, and daily prepareth himself to die."[4] Preparation for encountering the one St. Francis of Assisi called "Sister Death" has become a common monastic practice and is part of the wisdom traditions in many religions. To many twenty-first-century American minds, these medieval theological constructs might seem remote, impractical, or downright morbid, but many of the tenets of *Ars Moriendi* persist as wise advice in the present day, including informing the book that you are now reading. The daily meditation on one's own mortality found new life in the Croaker app, which five times every day sends a reminder that death is inevitable. The basic practical point, one that we have repeatedly iterated, is that the dignified and peaceful end of life that most of us desire requires preparation. And the essential first step in that preparation is honest consideration of our own death.

Dr. Linda Emanuel has termed the ability to face mortality "existential maturity."[5] She makes clear that there is no right or wrong way to achieve this and recognizes that acquisition of this state can develop gradually or occur in fits and starts. She says that existential maturity, in addition to empowering people to make informed choices and plans for the end of their lives, enhances the ability to live in a loving and meaningful way even when life is difficult. But, if it is such a good thing to envision one's dying and plan for it, how does one actually go about it?

HOW CAN I ENVISION MY DEATH?

Philosophical, theological, and psychological underpinnings of death awareness, such as those I've written about, interest me and other introspective and contemplative types and can provide fertile fields for research, but they are peripheral to the primary task: thinking about and planning for your own death. So, how do you start to honestly think about your own death, to encounter this foreign territory without getting frightened away or bogged down in morbid rumination on one hand or trivial clichés on the other? There is no wrong approach here, except, of course, for the one used by most Americans—to ignore death altogether and pretend it won't happen. But if you've made it this far in this book, you've already avoided that pitfall. What follows are actions that many have found helpful. I list them in two sections: "imaginings and ideas" are ways to identify and explore one's own values and feelings when it comes to dying, and "actions and advocacy" discusses practical tasks to accomplish.

In his superb book *The Five Invitations*, Frank Ostaseski, cofounder of the Zen Hospice Project, outlines and encourages a pentad of actions, practical steps for envisioning and encountering death that also result in living more fully. His first invitation, the one essential to the process, is simple but obvious: "Don't wait."[6]

Imaginings and Ideas

What is your favorite movie? Love song? Opera? Novel? Why do you like it? How does it touch you? Have you ever read a poem or heard a piece of music and thought, "That would be great to have performed at my funeral"? What was it about that selection that led you to the idea of your memorial service? It probably wasn't a catchy tune or a witty play on words; perhaps it was a memory or feeling it evoked, something that resonated deeply inside you. What aspect of that composition expressed an essential piece of who you are? What did that work say that you would like to communicate to those who care enough about you to show up at your service?

Did you ever, maybe after visiting a friend or relative in a hospital, silently say, "I sure hope nobody ever puts me through that" or "I'd rather just die than be kept alive that way"? Or perhaps you have attended a memorial service and thought that the proceedings were excessively morbid or, alternatively, celebratory to the point of denying grief, or irrelevant to who the departed one was for you? What was missing? What part of you found this distasteful?

These surprising encounters with emotions can be revelatory in that they expose or clarify a focal point of significance in the amorphous jumble of feelings we all carry around. If we pay attention to them, they can help us probe personal depths, the hidden parts of ourselves. When you have an experience like this, note your responses and ideas, maybe write them down so that later you can come back to them and contemplate what they tell you about yourself. Often, after people experience a meaningful funeral for a person who has had a dignified death or, less often, after witnessing someone suffering needlessly, dying in pain, they use these responses to inform their own choices and then incorporate them as they execute their own advance directives.[7]

These kinds of experiences can be catalysts as you imagine your end; more than transient thoughts, these responses and emotions expose important values you didn't realize you carried, values worth exploring as you think about your own dying and worth incorporating in your decisions. Take note of them, approach them in a mindful way, and record them somewhere when they occur; thoughts and feelings are notoriously fleeting.

Another useful source of images, thoughts, and feelings about the end of life is the rich trove of literature that explores and explains the world of the dying and of those who care for them. Each of us has our own style preferences, the types of stories that appeal to us, so I hesitate a bit to make strong recommendations, though the bibliography section of this book includes several thought-stimulating resources that I, and others, have found helpful.

Don't Forget You're Still Alive

Crazy as the thought may initially seem, envisioning one's death is often the easy part. Dying is a process, occasionally very brief but usually a more protracted experience characterized by variable rates of declining function and intensity of symptoms or suffering. In other words, dying is part of living, and thinking of ourselves as frail, with pain, weakening, and increasingly dependent is usually more threatening than imagining ourselves as absent. When you did the exercise in chapter 7, you encountered emotions that arose as you contemplated the progressive loss of everything and everyone, the process of dying. Use those feelings as grist as you grind through thoughts of your future final days. One way to process them is in the context of probing questions. There is a list of discussion questions at the back of this volume to assist in your thinking and talking about the end of your life.

What are you afraid of? Can you identify one thing that scares you more than anything else? Maybe look back at the list of common fears from chapter 6. Are you afraid of dying? What about it scares you? Are you afraid that you will suffer more than you are able to bear? What have you done in the past, when you felt afraid, that seemed to help? How might you use those resources now? Do you need to develop them further or find new sources of strength?

What will you hope for when you reach the point of knowing death is imminent? If you are facing this right now, is there a significant event you want to stay alive for? Are there things you know you should do or regret not having done? Is it more important to live longer even if much of that time is taken up with medical procedures and recovering from treatments? Or is your goal to focus on making the time you have left as much like you would want it to be as possible?

What are you willing to give up in order to live longer? What trade-offs are unacceptable? Undergoing medical treatment inevitably involves sacrifice. Sometimes these are physical things like an amputated leg or placement of a colostomy bag; sometimes they are less obvious, like having to give up smoking or eating foods you like. Are you willing to put up with side effects of a new treatment? Every medical treatment takes time, time that is the stuff of life, how life is usually measured; each loss or waste of time means less life left. How much time for treatment and side effects are you willing to cede in the hope of a longer life? Is it okay to postpone or cancel a planned family vacation so that you can get your medical treatments? Would you be willing to go on a breathing machine or other life-support device if it might keep you alive longer? If your family wanted you to take treatments you would rather not undergo, how important is it to keep them happy? Have you ever been in a situation that you found totally unacceptable? What was it that made it intolerable? What have you done, or what can you do, to make sure that that kind of thing never happens to you again?

Don't Go It Alone

While personal contemplation, as we have been describing, is tremendously useful in sorting out one's own thoughts and feelings, conversation often generates additional ideas and helps clarify amorphous or confusing imaginings. Talking with friends and family members, especially those who might be asked to speak for you at some time, is of particular value, though these conversations can be difficult to start. Many local hospices, senior centers, civic organizations, and faith communities sponsor groups or forums where people who are facing similar choices or difficulties, or who are at least open to listening and discussion, can meet, learn, and share.

A great place to help get conversations started is The Conversation Project,[8] where starter kits and numerous resources are available in several languages and are easy to download and/or print without charge. Another national organization, Death Cafes, promotes the process of people getting together over food (especially cake!) to talk about death and dying. There is no mandatory subject matter or perspective, just the willingness to eat and talk. Their mission is simple, and their website is easy to navigate.[9] Attending any one of these types of events or groups, especially with a family member or good friend, might be just what is needed for many people to clarify their own thoughts and desires.

Actions and Advocacy: Advance Care Planning

How can someone turn their envisioning into reality? This is the point of advance care planning. We presented this idea in chapter 2, primarily to introduce advance directives. But there are many more components to living your final days than just your medical care. There are several actions that, if taken now, can make a big difference in the way events occur.

Know the Rules

Does your health insurance plan cover hospice care, and are there any limits to coverage? Fortunately, problems in this area have become rare in most parts of the country, though they still exist. If you live in a care facility, what policies are in place that might impact your choices in the future? Does the facility have a contract with a hospice agency that would limit your options? Do they take a position on starting or stopping tube feeding? Does your faith community or clergy espouse or prohibit particular choices? Do you reside in a state that has legalized medical aid in dying?

Make Plans for Your Body's Disposition

Advance planning for your funeral or memorial service, choosing readings and songs, and selecting speakers (including talking with them about why you have selected them) is a tremendous gift for your surviving loved ones and ensures that your service speaks of who you are. If you also prepay the costs, this makes doubly sure that your wishes will be carried out. Most funeral directors provide this type of anticipatory guidance and arrangements.

Part of those arrangements entail disposition of your physical remains. The traditional American viewing of an embalmed corpse, followed by funeral service and cemetery burial, still occurs frequently, but alternatives such as cremation, body donation, "green burial," and even composting are increasingly used. Note that in most jurisdictions, if you wish to donate your body to a medical school or for research, you must act while you are still alive; donation of your organs or tissues for transplantation or other medical use usually requires action by your survivors, even if you have identified yourself as an organ and tissue donor. Several of the items in the bibliography at the end of this book include details and advice on these choices; for readers with more of a fascination in the fate of physical remains, the books *Stiff* by Mary Roach (2003) and *After We Die* by Norman L. Cantor (2010) provide entertaining and informative, if at times gruesome, reading.

Make Arrangements for Your "Stuff"

Even if you have few possessions, you need a will to clarify and ensure what will happen to them after you are gone. We all know we should do this, but we tend to procrastinate. Estate planning does not have to be complicated, though if your assets are large or complex, or if you have numerous survivors or specific bequests to make, working with an attorney is a good idea (and most lawyers will also assist in the completion of advance directives at the same time). Of course, having everything down on paper does not ensure that your family will not fight over the money or the "stuff" after you die, but, if they do, well, that's not your problem. After all, you won't be there anymore.

Part of your planning should include designating an "attorney in fact," someone who is authorized to perform business-related transactions on your behalf. The document that establishes this is called a power of attorney but differs from a Durable Power of Attorney for Health Care, as it deals with financial and business questions rather than those of medical care. The persons you designate to act for you in these two documents can be the same or different; it is totally up to you.

Do Your Medical Advance Care Planning

Advance directives (AD), detailed in chapter 2, are legally enforceable communications of one's preferences for care at the end of life. They come into play if you are not able to speak for yourself. In most states, execution of AD documents does not require an attorney, though most jurisdictions require witnesses or notarization to be legally enforceable. Forms for completion of AD are available from your doctor or attorney, from many social agencies, and online from various organizations, including the American Association of Retired Persons. The primary advance directives to complete include a living will, a document that communicates your preferences for care if you are terminally ill or in a persistent comatose state, and a Durable Power of Attorney for Health Care, in which you designate a specific person as having legal authority to speak on your behalf regarding medical decisions when you are unable to speak for yourself.

Another document to consider, depending on your situation, is a portable "do not resuscitate" (DNR) order, a legal form, signed by your physician, stating that in the event your breathing and/or heart stop functioning, CPR should not be started and every effort should be made to make you comfortable. Many states now also enforce Physician Orders for Life Sustaining Therapy (POLST), a document that anticipates several common medical scenarios and identifies your preferences for each, which are then signed as medical orders by your doctor.

Completing these documents in a way that accurately reflects your wishes is the single most important action you can take to increase the likelihood that the final period of your life corresponds to the image that you envision.

Make a Dignified Ending

Back in chapter 1, we identified the "five things of relationship completion," the statements that virtually all of us need to share with at least one person: "Forgive me," "I forgive you," "Thank you," "I love you," and "Good-bye." Think of those people who you need to say these things to, and then say them. Some of these people will be close to you, some may be from your distant past, some deceased. It may be uncomfortable to say or to hear these statements, but their communication almost always produces some healing and completion.

Every story has an ending; in many stories, the ending is what pulls together the meaning of the entire narrative. Many people facing the ending of their personal story are able to focus on what is vital and figure out something about what their life's significance was and is. In the *Bhagavad Gita*, Krishna says that "because death stirs people to seek answers to important spiritual questions, it becomes the greatest servant of humanity, rather than its most feared enemy."[10] Your story is your legacy, that part of you that you leave behind. Legacy work is a major concern of dignity therapy, as it helps focus on who you are and what is important.

When it comes to communicating a meaningful legacy, the method is much less important than the message. There are many ways of telling your story. Some people put together a scrapbook or arrange photograph albums. Many families celebrate the life of the departed one with a montage of photographs at a viewing or funeral; assisting in choosing those shots that will be shown helps you communicate who you are and what was important in your life, provides a structure for reflection on your life, and is a generous gift for your survivors. Other people write letters or otherwise leave messages to their children or grandchildren, even to those who have not yet been born. With the ubiquity of video technology on smartphones, it is simple to leave a video message, either something you create on your own or with the help of a family member or close friend who interviews you and records the conversation. Many hospice agencies can assist in producing and editing these written or recorded pieces of your legacy.

Make a Difference for the Future

As you have contemplated your ideas for the ending of your life, did you encounter roadblocks; frustrations with people, systems, or laws; or something that seemed to get in the way of your ability to envision and then enact your choices? Are any of these issues that, as part of your legacy, you would like to do something about? Maybe you thought about taking a more active role in your dying, like employing MAID, but that is not legal where you live. You might want to write your story for a newspaper or blog, or maybe communicate your frustration with legislators. You could get involved with an advocacy group, like Compassion and Choices. Or maybe you feel exactly the opposite, that life is so precious that nobody should take it away, even the person living it. Again, your story is a potent message that deserves to be heard.

ADVICE FOR COMPANIONS ON THE JOURNEY

Most people find it difficult, even painful, to be present with someone who is dying. The near-universal uncertainties are "What should I do?" and "I have no idea what to say." The short answer is that the words and actions are much less important than your presence. But here are a few practical comments.

Ask what you can do to help. Most people are hesitant to ask for help, but offer anyway. And mean it; don't ask if you're not going to act. If the patient won't give you a request, ask their family. Or maybe just look around the house; if you know the patient prided themselves on tidiness and the house is cluttered or dusty, ask if you can straighten up a bit or arrange to come back and clean. Baking pies or casseroles is an old-style act of comfort but is still a welcome gift, presuming you can cook. Asking ahead is good, as food that has to be discarded creates guilt along with the gratitude.

You will also be a better companion, whether as a daily caregiver or an occasional visitor, if you have done your own death homework; if you've read this book you're off to a good start. You already know that it is better to listen than to talk. If the suffering one asks for your advice, it is usually better to respond with another question than to tell them what to do. Rather than say, "Well, I think I would . . ." maybe try telling the story of something that helped you in a difficult situation—your faith, a wise conversation, a book or film—and leave it at that. Don't push your agenda.

In the ancient Hebrew story of Job, a man who suffered devastating losses and a chronic, painful, and disfiguring illness, we meet a group of his friends who came to provide comfort. If you know the story, you know that all the advice they gave only made this worse. But they did one thing right that usually gets overlooked. Their first response was to weep with Job, and then "they sat with him on the ground seven days and seven nights, and no one spoke a word to him, for they saw that his suffering was very great." [11] Most of us think that we understand things better that we actually do, that our advice has particular relevance and benefits. We are uncomfortable with suffering and want to fix things. But that is almost always the wrong thing to do. The primary gift you can give to someone facing any critical problem, especially someone facing the end of life, is your presence. The best message is "I am here."

ALLAN

I was astounded by the vigorous man I encountered at Allan's next appointment. He was off oxygen, his appetite and strength had returned, and he had begun running again. This was the most dramatic cancer treatment response that I ever witnessed. In the intervening years we have discovered more about how these new drugs, called targeted agents, work and how best to predict which patients will benefit, but for Allan, this seemed nothing short of a miraculous intervention. He lived another eighteen months or so. He returned to work and to service. The cancer eventually recurred in his brain, ending his life, but it never stole his breath again.

During this year-and-a-half respite, Allan was honored for distinguished service by a national organization supporting higher education. In his acceptance remarks, he challenged his audience: "If you're planning to do something distinguished, you'd better saddle up, because you're burning daylight."

9

WHAT'S IT ALL ABOUT, ANYWAY?

Death is an endless night so awful to contemplate that it can make us love life and value it with such passion that it may be the ultimate cause of all joy and all art.

—Paul Theroux

That October Friday dawned a bit cold, but the crispness in the air promised a delightful day to come. Debbie left home early; she had paperwork to finish before the hospice interdisciplinary team meeting at eight o'clock. She kissed Adam on her way out the door, reminding him to deliver the kids to school on time, with teeth brushed and lunches packed. The team meeting was well underway when Debbie was called away; Adam had been in an accident and needed her to meet him at the emergency room.

The morning sun glared in her rearview mirror as she drove to the hospital. "That Adam! He can't sit still for an hour and now he'll be in some kind of cast and I'll have to do everything for him; and I'll tease him, and he'll hate it all." She was still chuckling nervously as she exited her car and walked to the hospital door. But there would be no cast, no doing everything for him, no teasing. He lay in solitude, his body partially covered by a sheet, the detritus of the failed resuscitation efforts littering the cubicle. When she touched the cloth that covered the upper part of his face, she felt a gooey clotted mass where his forehead should have been.

Debbie was one of the best nurses I ever worked with. She was caring and competent, insightful and industrious. She had a bedside presence that put even the most anxious daughter or irascible old codger at ease, exuding the sense that here was a nurse who knew what she was doing, who cared about them, and who would spare no energy to accomplish what was needed. Without Adam, though, Debbie might never have become that exceptional nurse.

Debbie's abusive childhood and troubled adolescence left her with difficulty acknowledging her value and accepting that she could be loved. A religious conversion experience gave her a new outlook, and a month later she met Adam. Six years her senior, he was the owner of an agricultural services business, supplying farmers with seed and fertilizer, part of the lifeblood of the rural Ohio community and economy. Adam, smitten but not blind, recognized Debbie's pain, saw both that it would take time for her to grow to love and be loved and that his passion for her could be part of that healing. They met in June and were married in December.

With the start of a family, Debbie immersed herself in the busyness of raising toddlers, developing homemaker skills, and becoming an active member of her church and community. But she sensed a need for something more. Adam had once told her, "You're not only special; you're able to accomplish anything you want to accomplish." One day she mentioned a long-standing whim about being a nurse; he encouraged her to check out all the nursing schools within a fifty-mile radius and get on with it. She described him as "one of those 'push' kind of guys." He pushed himself too, farming his own land in addition to running the business, and he was respected and successful at both.

IS THERE MEANING IN DEATH?

We treat death with both respect and avoidance. We see dying, whether our own or that of one we love, as both intimate and alien. We treat corpses with peculiar dignity, dress them in finery, and surround them with flowers. We have developed rituals and ceremonies for the disposal of the remains and for saying good-bye to the person who once inhabited them. These practices allow us to both approach and remain detached from the reality of mortality.

When we attend a wake, funeral, or memorial event, our emotions and memories resonate, often very deeply, witnessing to the importance of what we are doing. We perceive that something consequential is occurring in this final acknowledgment of a life. But what exactly does it mean? What is the point? Does death mean anything at all beyond the cessation of biological existence? In the infinity of the cosmos, does the dying of a human being matter any more than the pulling of a weed in the garden? Is our attitude toward mortality nothing more than instinct for survival of the species? Or is human demise somehow of consequence?

These are not new questions. In the ancient Hebrew wisdom book of Ecclesiastes, an author called "the Teacher" recounts and comments on what he has observed and experienced during his lifelong search for the meaning of life. He posed it this way: "For the fate of humans and the fate of animals is the same; as one dies, so dies the other. They all have the same breath, and humans have no advantage over the animals; for all is vanity. All go to one place; all are from the dust, and all turn to dust again."[1]

But most of us don't really buy that idea, do we? We think we're somehow special, that human beings are somehow different from other animals. We consider ourselves as unique individuals; we think in terms of personhood, of human rights. We feel infinitely superior to the gnat buzzing around us. And if the human species is of greater value, then a human death is also of more significance than the swatting of an insect.

Our philosophic and religious traditions support this hierarchy. Many Eastern traditions acknowledge all sentient life as of value but still view existence in humans, as opposed to "lower" forms, as more propitious. Western monotheistic traditions posit humanity as uniquely "created in the image of God." Roman Catholic teaching boldly states that all human life is sacred, from the moment of conception to the time of natural death.

Do we differ from slugs only by our DNA? If so, then death simply completes a biologic cycle, makes room for more of our species, and creates fertilizer for the earth. Or are we connected with all other beings in a universal consciousness? If so, when we die, we continue the cycles of suffering and rebirth, straining toward enlightenment and becoming unified with the cosmos. Or could it be that we are uniquely endowed with a spark of divinity? If so, then our death is a precious and profound event. The Teacher in Ecclesiastes put it well: "Who knows?"

ADAM AND DYING

Like every farm boy, Adam was acquainted with death. It became personal when he was twenty years old; his older brother parked some farm equipment in contact with a power line and was electrocuted. His younger brother suffered from an ill-defined autoimmune disease that damaged organ after organ and eventually cost him his life. Just a month before he met Debbie, one of Adam's employees, applying anhydrous ammonia to a hilly cornfield, rolled the tractor and was asphyxiated by the fumes.

Debbie said that the deaths of so many young men close to him gave Adam an awareness of the fragility of life. In his practical nature, he made arrangements for the sale of his company in the event of his demise. He referred to Debbie's nursing degree as their "insurance policy." He thought about his funeral and listed the songs he wanted used at the service in the front pages of his Bible. Debbie said this kind of talk freaked her out at first, but their relationship developed such that talking about their deaths, while not constant and never morbid, became something very easy for them to do.

RANDOMNESS

When death appears random, like Adam's, where do we find the meaning? Our minds search for significance, a pattern, a purpose; we rebel at the thought that something so personally threatening as our own mortality might occur at the whim of the cosmos.

Our parents taught us that actions have consequences. So, when we suffer what we see as consequences, we look for causes, especially in our previous actions. Religious traditions support the idea that our lives are affected by forces outside ourselves and that judgment is part of that equation. One of the basic tenets of Buddhism is that every event has a cause (or causes). The cause may be obvious, like the lung cancer that develops in a three-pack-a-day smoker, or it may be obscure or remote, even stemming from a previous life, but it is there. This idea, part of the concept of karma, resonates strongly with our collective sense of justice. The theology of the ancient Hebrews imagined living and dying as part of a divine reward and punishment system. The Psalms are filled with prayers for God to strike the wicked. The stories in the Torah and the Prophets repeatedly show God acting to destroy those who disobey or rebel. The converse, that faithfulness results in longevity, is also ubiquitous. In the book of Proverbs, both parts are spelled out: "The fear of the Lord prolongs life, but the years of the wicked will be cut short."[2]

The problem, though, is that human experience shows that it doesn't work that way. Virtuous young men are killed in battle, while perpetrators of Nazi atrocities live comfortably to old age in South America. Corrupt politicians enjoy their power and lucre, seemingly impervious to any consequences, and young fathers die in truck accidents. Faced with these events that fly in the face of our vision of a just God or a moral universe, we survive by chalking it up as something we can't understand, explain it away with clichés. Often, we pull out platitudes like "God moves in mysterious ways" or "At least they're not suffering anymore." But these are simply other ways to say that we have no idea why what is happening has occurred. The Teacher of Ecclesiastes noted it this way: "In my vain life I have seen everything; there are righteous people who perish in their righteousness, and there are wicked people who prolong their life in their evildoing."[3]

Conversations that occur at hospice bedsides and in funeral parlors demonstrate that we search for meaning even when there seems to be none. The number of times that I heard a terminally ill patient ask, "Why me? What did I do to deserve this?" indicates that this search is virtually universal. We Americans seem to accept the idea of "the luck of the draw" when it comes to deaths from accidents and natural disasters, though news reports of these events usually include speculation into who might be to blame. This whole, bigger question of why "bad things happen to good people" has been the subject of countless philosophical and theological manuscripts, Sunday School class discussions, and wake conversations. Perusing the religion section at a bookstore reveals how much this question has been a boon to the publishing industry and to authors who thought they had some novel idea about the topic. But it has pretty much all been said before; our friend, the Teacher, said, "There is nothing new under the sun."[4]

When Jesus was asked about this, he alluded to a recent tragedy near Jerusalem, where a tower had collapsed and crushed eighteen people to death. Jesus said that there was nothing particularly evil or righteous about the casualties; they were just in the wrong place at the wrong time.[5] That's just the way it is. That's the way the world works. There was no overriding meaning in the timing of their deaths. Put in twenty-first-century terminology, what he was saying was, "Hey, stuff happens."

DEBBIE'S PERSPECTIVE

When Debbie reflected on what Adam's death meant, her first thought was about seat belts. He was an independent sort, naturally fighting back against anything that seemed restraining, even refusing to wear a seat belt when driving. They had a running joke about this; the first new car they bought together came with a promotion from General Motors that paid $10,000 to the survivors of anyone who died in a motor vehicle accident while wearing their seat belt in that car. So, when the family loaded up for a ride, they buckled up together, chiming in unison, "Ten thousand dollars!" That Friday morning, after he dropped the children off at school, Adam continued with a truckload of soybeans to the grain elevator. Going around a curve, he lost control and the truck rolled several times. Even after landing upside down, the truck was basically intact, so if Adam had been buckled in, he likely would have survived. Debbie's twin sister told her that she was angry with Adam because he never wanted to wear a seat belt. Debbie replied, "I'm just going to let you be angry about this, because I can't. I cannot be angry with Adam for dying. It just doesn't make sense."

But then as she was telling me her story, Debbie reflected on Adam's calling hours, the number of people who showed up, many of whom said that Adam's dying had awakened them to be a better husband, wife, child, farmer, businessman, nurse, Christian, person. She knew that most of those promises would never be kept, most of those new leaves never turned over, but she recognized that Adam and his death had affected the community of people around them. She said, "I really felt at the time that there was a purpose for his death. I knew there was a purpose for his life." Would she have married him if she knew he would die, knew she would be a widow at thirty-two? Absolutely. "I wouldn't have been the woman that I was without him, because he taught me how to be a decent human being and to stop the cycle of how I was raised. So, I think that if, well, if that was the only time I could have with him, I was okay with that."

DEATH INFORMS LIFE INFORMS DEATH

Could it be that there is a clue in what Debbie said? From Adam's perspective, his death was a tragic but accidental event, a wrong place and wrong time scenario. But for Debbie, it was the revelation of all that Adam had been for her and for seemingly countless others. Maybe if death has any meaning, it is imbued by the life that led up to it. It seems axiomatic that if human death has significance, it must somehow be tied up with the meaning or meaningfulness of life. If life is just a cosmic accident, then death must be equally absurd. But if life, the life of one's self or that of a loved one, has identifiable personal meaning and purpose, then its ending must also have individual significance. The existence of meaning in the death of any person is dependent on the meaning of the existence that preceded it. If this is true, then any meaning of dying must be found at the individual level and that searching for some universal purpose is doomed to futility.

But Debbie's observations raise an even deeper truth. Adam's life and death achieved significance because he lived that life in relationship with others. His love healed his wife and nurtured his children. His forthrightness attracted his friends and encouraged his customers and colleagues. His dying produced a vacuum that delineated his substance for every person who knew him.

When we consider our own impending deaths, they appear profoundly meaningful; in contrast, when the deaths of others look random or remote, they exude little substance and can even seem absurd. Our search for the overall meaning of death leads to a paradox of consequential absurdity. Because dying happens to everyone, it is commonplace and of little significance; because it happens to me, it is of ultimate importance.

Is there, then, some practical bottom line in this pondering of the meaning of death? It seems to me that it is also summed up in a paradox: learning how to die is the best way to learn how to live. And, as Adam taught us, for our lives and deaths to grow in significance, they must be lived in relationship with others, for it is only they who will recognize the meaning after we are gone. It was at this pragmatic level that the Teacher finally found his conclusions: "Go, eat your bread with enjoyment, and drink your wine with a merry heart. . . . Enjoy life with the wife whom you love, all the days of your vain life that are given you under the sun, because that is your portion in life."[6]

So, what if death itself has no overarching meaning beyond the ending of biological existence? What if, despite the rituals and emotions, the dogmas and philosophies, there is no overriding significance to the ending of a human life? Everything we have looked at has declared the same message: death may be nothing, but life is everything; and to make life complete, the one living the life must continue living until the end. Knowing that we will die can instruct us in how to live well, and living well increases the likelihood of dying well.

❋ ❋ ❋

Adam was to have received an award from the local soil and water conservation board. Debbie attended the meeting, only a month after her husband's funeral, to accept the honor on his behalf. She met an elderly woman sitting near her who recognized who she was. Debbie describes the encounter this way:

> And she says to me, "Oh, you're the Simpson widow." I feel like my skin is wrinkling as she spoke it. And so, I said, "Yeah, I am." And she said, "You know, I lost my husband two years ago, and I'm still angry at him because there's still a lot I don't know." And I sat there, and I thought, "What a horrible place to be. . . . Sure, I'm mad as hell that I don't have the husband that I thought I'd grow old with, and we had more that we wanted to do, but I'm glad I didn't have any more questions.
>
> And it's funny, because the obituary, you know, blah, blah, blah, married Debbie Ames, and then it says, "She survives." And I said to somebody a few days later, "I know I'm going to get through this because it says in the paper that I survived."

❋ ❋ ❋

A statement that particularly irritates me is when I read in an obituary that someone "lost their battle with . . ." This is a tragic sentiment. In my career of caring for patients with cancer and those dying from every disease imaginable, I have met very few who "lost the battle." Sure, the cancer, heart failure, lung disease, dementia, or other fatal medical condition caused them to die. But the only ones who lose the battle are those who concede, who "give up," who allow the disease or the dying to deprive them of the essence of who they are. Concession takes multiple forms, but what characterizes all giving up is misunderstanding what you are fighting for and what is staked on the outcome. Continuing to scratch for yet one more magic treatment to wipe out the disease that is attacking you might fit with who you are, but more often it represents blindness to reality. Recognizing that a disease is going to cause your body to die is not giving up; it is honestly facing the enemy. Your body is only one weapon you have in your fight and only one part of what you risk losing. Your character, values, emotions, will, and the support of those close to you are equally important. The disease might kill you, but it cannot stop you from living. Allan lived as fully while he was dying as he did when he was healthy and in his interregnum. In chapter 7, I told the story of my father's cardiac arrest. He lived for eight years after that event, always aware that death could be imminent. Having faced death made it easier for him to live. It is a profound truth that knowing that life is limited, that it will end, increases its value.

Admitting that you are going to die and making plans for it is not conceding. In fact, it is perhaps the wisest battle plan. It takes courage and honesty to imagine your own death, to make preparations for it. After you do these things, death becomes less frightening. You can then focus on living. As we've seen repeatedly, that's the whole point anyway.

I started this book with Socrates on trial, awaiting condemnation by the Athenian court, knowing he would die soon. As he had expected, he was found guilty and sentenced to execution. His farewell message was, "Well, now it is time to be off, I to die and you to live; but which of us has the happier prospect is unknown to anyone but God."[7]

ACKNOWLEDGMENTS

I am indebted to innumerable family members, friends, and colleagues for their encouragement, suggestions, and ideas. I notably thank the Rev. Dr. Amy Greene for her understanding of religious and spiritual pain and its relief, and the Rev. Chuck Behrens for his insight into the fears of the dying and for being a wise sounding board. Fauzia Burke of FSB Associates is a kindhearted but demanding publicist and coach as well as the source of the final title. At the Rudy Agency, Maryann Karinch saw something in my work that convinced her this novice writer had a chance, and Lauren Manoy took me under her wing with cogent advice, reassurance, and a bit of prodding to get the manuscript tuned and submitted. Suzanne Staszak-Silva and Janice Braunstein at Rowman & Littlefield saw something of value in my work and shaped my rambling syntax into a readable book. To Pat, my wife and soulmate for the past thirty-five years, your inspiration, support, and love keep me going. My greatest debt, though, is to the hundreds of patients whose lives and stories have touched mine. I only hope my efforts on your behalf can serve as partial repayment of all that you taught and gave me. Thank you.

DISCUSSION QUESTIONS

INTRODUCTION

1. What do you think happens when we die? Where did those ideas come from?
2. Tell the story of the death of someone close to you.

CHAPTER 1: DYING IN AMERICA

1. Would you rather die unexpectedly and suddenly or know it was coming and have time to prepare? Why?
2. What would a good death look like for you?
3. If you knew you were dying, who would you need to communicate a final message to?

CHAPTER 2: I'M GOING TO DIE? WHAT CAN I DO?

1. You are dying. There is no way to avoid it. How does that knowledge make you feel?
2. Have you ever had to make a medical decision for someone else? How did that make you feel?

3. Do you have advance directives in place? Have you talked about your preferences with the person you want to speak for you?
4. If you were unable to eat or drink, would you want tube feedings? Why or why not?
5. In the story about Madeline, did Lucita provide comfort or violate Madeline's wishes?

CHAPTER 3: HOSPICE

1. Have you had experience with hospice care? What was good or bad about it?
2. What do you think about the requirement that patients abandon coverage for most disease-directed treatment in order to obtain the Medicare Hospice Benefit?
3. Have you or someone you know received palliative care?

CHAPTER 4: SUFFERING

1. Describe the differences between "pain" and "suffering."
2. How does our culture teach us to suffer "in silence"?
3. Can you imagine a situation in which you would rather die than continue to endure what you were experiencing?
4. Do you think there is an ethical line between relieving suffering and hastening death that should not be crossed? Where would you draw that line? Where should the law draw that line?
5. Is there a difference between suffering caused by physical symptoms and that produced by emotional distress?

CHAPTER 5: IT'S MY LIFE, ISN'T IT?

1. Describe a real or hypothetical end-of-life care situation. How do the principles of beneficence, nonmaleficence, justice, and autonomy affect the decisions a patient makes? What about a doctor's decisions?
2. Brittany Maynard's public story generated extensive interest and reaction. What do you think about her decision and rationale?
3. What limits should there be on people dying "on their own terms"?
4. To whom or what have you ceded partial control over your life? What impact will they have on decisions you make when you are dying?
5. How does the government's responsibility to preserve life affect an individual's ability to make their own life and death decisions?

CHAPTER 6: WHAT'S GOD GOT TO DO WITH IT?

1. When you think about dying, what frightens you?
2. What does spirituality mean to you?
3. How does your belief system inform your thoughts about dying?
4. Is there a relationship between behavior and subsequent suffering?
5. How can there be hope in death?

CHAPTER 7: WHAT DOES IT FEEL LIKE TO DIE?

1. Have you known anyone who reported a "near-death" experience? How did they describe it? What do you think happened to them?

2. What item was most difficult for you to cross off your list? Why?
3. How did you feel when you crossed off the last item?

CHAPTER 8: ENVISIONING YOUR OWN DEATH

1. What does a dignified death look like?
2. What message or story about yourself do you want others to know after you are gone?
3. What would you like your funeral or memorial service to look like?

CHAPTER 9: WHAT'S IT ALL ABOUT, ANYWAY?

1. Write a paragraph about the meaning of your own death.

NOTES

INTRODUCTION

1. Plato, *The Last Days of Socrates*, trans. Hugh Tredennick and Harold Tarant (London: Penguin Books, 2003), 55.

2. Atul Gawande, *Being Mortal: Medicine and What Matters in the End* (New York: Metropolitan Books, 2014), 8.

3. Ahmed Ali, trans., *Al-Qur'ān: A Contemporary Translation* (Princeton, NJ: Princeton University Press, 1984), 467 (Sura 56, verse 60).

1. DYING IN AMERICA

1. Ira Byock, *Dying Well: The Prospect for Growth at the End of Life* (New York: Riverhead Books, 1997), 140.

2. Karen E. Steinhauser et al., "Factors Considered Important at the End of Life by Patients, Family, Physicians, and Other Care Providers," *Journal of the American Medical Association* 284 (2000): 2478, https://doi.org/10.1001/jama.284.19.2476.

3. Joan M. Teno et al., "Site of Death, Place of Care, and Health Care Transitions among US Medicare Beneficiaries, 2000–2015," *Journal of the American Medical Association* 320 (2018): 267, https://doi.org/10.1001/jama.2018.8981.

4. The SUPPORT Principal Investigators, "A Controlled Trial to Improve Care for Seriously Ill Hospitalized Patients: The Study to Understand Prognoses and Preferences for Outcomes and Risks of Treatments (SUPPORT)," *Journal of the American Medical Association* 274 (1995): 1593–95, https://doi.org/10.1001/jama.1995.03530200027032.

5. Jessica Nutik Zitter, *Extreme Measures: Finding a Better Path to the End of Life* (New York: Avery, 2017), 19ff.

6. Teno et al., "Site of Death, Place of Care, and Health Care Transitions among US Medicare Beneficiaries, 2000–2015."

2. I'M GOING TO DIE? WHAT CAN I DO?

1. Kenneth D. Kochanek, Sherry L. Murphy, Jiaquan Xu, and Elizabeth Arias, "Deaths: Final Data for 2017," *National Vital Statistics Reports* 68 (2019): 6, https://www.cdc.gov/nchs/data/nvsr/nvsr68/nvsr68_09-508.pdf.

2. Quoted in Atul Gawande, *Being Mortal: Medicine and What Matters in the End* (New York: Metropolitan Books, 2014), 182.

3. Erin S. DeMartino et al., "Who Decides When a Patient Can't? Statutes on Alternate Decision Makers," *New England Journal of Medicine* 376 (2017): 1479–81, https://doi.org/10.1056/NEJMms1611497.

4. Bryan McNally et al., "Out-of-Hospital Cardiac Arrest Surveillance—Cardiac Arrest Registry to Enhance Survival (CARES), United States, October 1, 2005–December 31, 2010," *Morbidity and Mortality Weekly Report Surveillance Summaries* 60 (2011): 11, https://www.cdc.gov/mmwr/preview/mmwrhtml/ss6008a1.htm?s_cid=ss6008a1_w.

5. POLST is the most commonly used acronym. Alternatives include POST (Physician Orders for Scope of Treatment), MOST (Medical Orders for Scope of Treatment), MOLST (Medical Orders for Life-Sustaining Treatment), and TPOPP (Transportable Physician Orders for Patient Preferences).

6. Susan Toll and Joan M. Teno, "Lessons from Oregon in Embracing Complexity in End-of-Life Care," *New England Journal of Medicine* 376 (2017): 1078–82, https://doi.org/10.1056/NEJMsb1612511.

7. Thomas E. Finucane, Colleen Christmas, and Kathy Travis, "Tube Feeding in Patients with Advanced Dementia: A Review of the Evi-

dence," *Journal of the American Medical Association* 282 (1999): 1365–70, https://doi.org/10.1001/jama.282.14.1365.

3. HOSPICE

1. Cecily E. Saunders, foreword to *Oxford Textbook of Palliative Medicine*, 3rd ed., ed. Derek Doyle, Geoffrey Hanks, Nathan Cherny, and Kenneth Calman (Oxford: Oxford University Press, 2004), xviii.
2. "Medicare and Medicaid Programs: Hospice Conditions of Participation," Department of Health and Human Services, June 5, 2008, https://www.govinfo.gov/content/pkg/FR-2008-06-05/pdf/08-1305.pdf.
3. Department of Health and Human Services, "Hospice Compare," accessed November 10, 2019, https://www.medicare.gov/hospicecompare.
4. Jennifer S. Temel et al., "Early Palliative Care for Patients with Metastatic Non-Small-Cell Lung Cancer," *New England Journal of Medicine* 363 (2010): 737–39, https://doi.org/10.1056/NEJMoa1000678.
5. American Society of Clinical Oncology, "Integration of Palliative Care into Standard Oncology Care: American Society of Clinical Oncology Practice Guideline Update," *Journal of Clinical Oncology* 35 (2017): 96–112, https://ascopubs.org/doi/10.1200/JCO.2016.70.1474.

4. SUFFERING

1. Eric J. Cassell, *The Nature of Suffering and the Goals of Medicine* (Oxford: Oxford University Press, 1991), 33.
2. Alphonse Daudet, *In the Land of Pain*, ed. and trans. Julian Barnes (New York: Alfred A. Knopf, 2002), 23.
3. Daudet, *In the Land of Pain*, 19.
4. Sebastiano Mercadente et al., "Controlled Sedation for Refractory Symptoms in Dying Patients," *Journal of Pain and Symptom Management* 37 (2009): 775, https://doi.org/10.1016/j.jpainsymman.2008.04.020.
5. Gary Cheung, Gwendolyn Douwes, and Frederick Sundram, "Late-Life Suicide in Terminal Cancer: A Rational Act or Underdiagnosed Depression?" *Journal of Pain and Symptom Management* 54 (2017): 837, https://doi.org/10.1016/j.jpainsymman.2017.05.004.

6. Linda Ganzini et al., "Nurses' Experiences with Hospice Patients Who Refuse Food and Fluids to Hasten Death," *New England Journal of Medicine* 349 (2003): 359–65, https://doi.org/10.1056/NEJMsa035086.

7. Brittany Maynard, "My Right to Death with Dignity at 29," (originally CNN), accessed November 10, 2019, https://compassionandchoices.org/stories/brittany-maynard/.

8. Many other terms have been applied to this procedure, most notably "physician-assisted suicide" and "death with dignity." I use the term "medical aid in dying" as a hopefully more neutral descriptive term.

9. "Oregon Revised Statute: Oregon's Death with Dignity Act," Oregon Health Authority, accessed November 10, 2019, https://www.oregon.gov/oha/PH/PROVIDERPARTNERRESOURCES/EVALUATIONRESEARCH/DEATHWITHDIGNITYACT/Pages/ors.aspx.

10. "Oregon Death with Dignity Act: 2018 Data Summary," Oregon Health Authority, accessed November 10, 2019, https://www.oregon.gov/oha/PH/PROVIDERPARTNERRESOURCES/EVALUATIONRESEARCH/DEATHWITHDIGNITYACT/Documents/year21.pdf.

11. Charles Blanke et al., "Characterizing 18 Years of the Death with Dignity Act in Oregon," *JAMA Oncology* 3 (2017): 1405, https://doi.org/10.1001/jamaoncol.2017.0243.

12. Veena Shankaran, Richard J. LaFrance, and Scott D. Ramsey, "Drug Price Inflation and the Cost of Assisted Death for Terminally Ill Patients—Death with Indignity," *JAMA Oncology* 3 (2017): 15, https://doi.org/10.1001/jamaoncol.2016.3842.

13. J. J. E. Koopman and H. Putter, "Regional Variation in the Practice of Euthanasia and Physician-Assisted Suicide in the Netherlands," *Netherlands Journal of Medicine* 74 (2016): 387–94, http://www.njmonline.nl/article.php?a=1777&d=1181&i=200.

14. Pauline S. C. Kouwenhoven et al., "Opinions about Euthanasia and Advanced Dementia: A Qualitative Study among Dutch Physicians and Members of the General Public," *BMC Medical Ethics* 16, no. 7 (2015): 2, https://doi.org/10.1186/1472-6939-16-7.

15. Cees D. M. Ruijs, Gerrit van der Wal, Ad J. F. M. Kerkhof, and Bregje D. Onwuteaka-Philipsen, "Unbearable Suffering and Requests for Euthanasia Prospectively Studied in End-of-Life Cancer Patients in

Primary Care," *BMC Palliative Care* 13 (2014): 5, https://doi.org/10. 1186/1472-684X-13-62.

16. Derek W. Braverman et al., "Health Care Professionals' Attitudes about Physician-Assisted Death: An Analysis of Their Justifications and the Roles of Terminology and Patient Competency," *Journal of Pain and Symptom Management* 54 (2017): 540–41, https://doi.org/10.1016/j. jpainsymman.2017.07.024.

17. Jack D. McCue, "Freud's Physician-Assisted Death," *Archives of Internal Medicine* 159 (1999): 1521, https://doi.org/10.1001/archinte.159. 14.1521.

5. IT'S MY LIFE, ISN'T IT?

1. Brittany Maynard, "My Right to Death with Dignity at 29" (originally CNN), accessed November 10, 2019, https:// compassionandchoices.org/stories/brittany-maynard.

2. Philip G. Johnson, "Raleigh Seminarian with Terminal Brain Cancer Responds to Brittany Maynard," Catholic Diocese of Raleigh, accessed November 10, 2019, https://dioceseofraleigh.org/news/raleigh-seminarian-terminal-brain-cancer-responds-brittany-maynard.

3. Maggie Karner, "Brain Cancer Will Likely Kill Me, but There's No Way I'll Kill Myself," TheFederalist.com, October 10, 2014, accessed November 10, 2019, https://thefederalist.com/2014/10/10/brain-cancer-will-likely-kill-me-but-theres-no-way-ill-kill-myself.

4. Genesis 2:24, New Revised Standard Version.

5. "A Brief Statement of Faith," 345, Presbyterian Church (USA), accessed November 10, 2019, http://oga.pcusa.org/site_media/media/uploads/oga/pdf/boc2016.pdf.

6. Lawrence O. Gostin, "Ethics, the Constitution, and the Dying Process: The Case of Theresa Marie Schiavo," *Journal of the American Medical Association* 293 (2005): 2404, https://doi.org/10.1001/jama.293. 19.2403.

6. WHAT'S GOD GOT TO DO WITH IT?

1. Mark 11:24, New Revised Standard Version (NRSV).

2. James 5:16b, NRSV.

3. James 5:13–15, NRSV.

4. John 11:25, NRSV.

5. Andrea C. Phelps et al., "Religious Coping and Use of Intensive Life-Prolonging Care Near Death in Patients with Advanced Cancer," *Journal of the American Medical Association* 301 (2009): 1140, https://doi.org/10.1001/jama.2009.341.

6. Lenworth M. Jacobs, Karyl Burns, and Barbara Bennett Jacobs, "Trauma Death: Views of the Public and Trauma Professionals on Death and Dying from Injuries," *Archives of Surgery* 143 (2008): 734, https://doi.org/10.1001/archsurg.143.8.730.

7. Phelps et al., "Religious Coping," 1144.

8. Michael J. Balboni et al., "U.S. Clergy Religious Values and Relationships to End-of-Life Discussions and Care," *Journal of Pain and Symptom Management* 53 (2017): 1001–4, https://doi.org/10.1016/j.jpainsymman.2016.12.346.

9. Melissa M. Garrido et al., "Pathways from Religion to Advance Care Planning: Beliefs about Control over Length of Life and End-of-Life Values," *Gerontologist* 53 (2013): 809, https://doi.org/10.1093/geront/gns128.

10. Job 14:5, NRSV.

11. Koran 3:145.

12. Ecclesiastes 9:5a, NRSV.

13. Gyurme Dorje, trans., *The Tibetan Book of the Dead*, ed. Graham Coleman with Thupten Jinpa (New York: Viking, 2005).

14. Luke 16:19–25, NRSV.

15. Matthew 27:46, NRSV.

16. Numbers 32:23b, NRSV.

17. Balboni et al., "U.S. Clergy Religious Values," 1001.

18. James 1:2–4, NRSV.

19. Samir Selmanovic, "If Muhammad Had Not Spoken," in *My Neighbor's Faith: Stories of Interreligious Encounter, Growth, and Transformation*, ed. Jennifer Howe Peace, Or N. Rose, and Gregory Mobley (Maryknoll, NY: Orbis Books, 2012), 211.

20. Krista Tippett, *Becoming Wise: An Inquiry into the Mystery and Art of Living* (New York: Penguin Books, 2016), 251.

7. WHAT DOES IT FEEL LIKE TO DIE?

1. Plato, *The Last Days of Socrates*, trans. Hugh Tredennick and Harold Tarant (London: Penguin Books, 2003), 69.

2. Plato, *The Republic*, trans. Benjamin Jowett (New York: Modern Library, 1941), Book X.

3. Job 10:22, New Revised Standard Version (NRSV).

4. Ahmed Ali, trans., *Al-Qur'ān: A Contemporary Translation* (Princeton, NJ: Princeton University Press, 1984), 14 (Sura 2, verse 25).

5. Ali, *Al-Qur'ān*, 252–53 (Sura 18, verse 29).

6. Gyurme Dorje, trans., *The Tibetan Book of the Dead*, ed. Graham Coleman with Thupten Jinpa (New York: Viking, 2005).

7. Mark Twain, *The Autobiography of Mark Twain* (New York: Harper & Row, 2010), 326–27.

8. John 14:3b, NRSV.

9. John Milton, *Paradise Lost* (New York: Oxford University Press, 2005), 307.

10. W. Y. Evans-Wentz, trans. and ed., *The Tibetan Book of the Dead* (London: Oxford University Press, 1927), 160–61.

11. https://drjeffspiess.com/images/jeffspiess/site/contents/Dying%20Without%20Distress%20Chapter%207%20Worksheet.pdf.

12. Leo Tolstoy, "The Death of Ivan Ilyich," in *The Death of Ivan Ilyich and Other Stories*, trans. Rosemary Edmonds (London: Penguin Books, 1960), 130.

13. Tolstoy, "The Death of Ivan Ilyich," 144.

14. Tolstoy, "The Death of Ivan Ilyich," 152.

15. Tolstoy, "The Death of Ivan Ilyich," 154.

8. ENVISIONING YOUR OWN DEATH

1. Mark Twain, *The Adventures of Tom Sawyer* (New York: Penguin, 2014), 115–17.

2. Harvey Max Chochinov et al., "The Effect of Dignity Therapy on Distress and End-of-Life Experience in Terminally Ill Patients: A Randomised Controlled Trial," *Lancet Oncology* 12 (2011): 754.

3. Psalm 116:15, New Revised Standard Version (NRSV).

4. Thomas à Kempis, *The Imitation of Christ* (New York: Grosset and Dunlap, 1973), 50.

5. Linda L. Emanuel et al., "'And Yet It Was a Blessing': The Case for Existential Maturity," *Journal of Palliative Medicine* 20 (2017): 319.

6. Frank Ostaseski, *The Five Invitations: Discovering What Death Can Teach Us about Living Fully* (New York: Flat Iron Books, 2017), 15.

7. Deborah Carr, "'I Don't Want to Die Like That . . .': The Impact of Significant Others' Death Quality on Advance Care Planning," *Gerontologist* 52 (2012): 774.

8. The Conversation Project, "Starter Kits," accessed November 20, 2019, https://www.theconversationproject.org/starter-kits.

9. Death Cafe, accessed November 20, 2019, https://deathcafe.com.

10. Jack Hawley, *The Bhagavad Gita: A Walkthrough for Westerners* (Novato, CA: New World Library, 2001): 73–74.

11. Job 2:13, NRSV.

9. WHAT'S IT ALL ABOUT, ANYWAY?

1. Ecclesiastes 3:19–20, New Revised Standard Version (NRSV).

2. Proverbs 10:27, NRSV.

3. Ecclesiastes 7:15, NRSV.

4. Ecclesiastes 1:9, NRSV.

5. Luke 13:4–5, NRSV.

6. Ecclesiastes 9:7–10, NRSV.

7. Plato, *The Last Days of Socrates*, trans. Hugh Tredennick and Harold Tarant (London: Penguin Books, 2003), 70.

BIBLIOGRAPHY

Ali, Ahmed, trans. *Al-Qur'ān: A Contemporary Translation*. Princeton, NJ: Princeton University Press, 1984.

American Society of Clinical Oncology. "Integration of Palliative Care into Standard Oncology Care." Published online October 31, 2016. https://ascopubs.org/doi/10.1200/JCO.2016.70.1474.

Balboni, Michael J., Adam Sullivan, Andrea C. Enzinger, Patrick T. Smith, Christine Mitchell, John R. Peteet, James A. Tulsky, Tyler VanderWeele, and Tracy A. Balboni. "U.S. Clergy Religious Values and Relationships to End-of-Life Discussions and Care." *Journal of Pain and Symptom Management* 53 (2017): 999–1008. https://doi.org/10.1016/j.jpainsymman.2016.12.346.

Beard, Richard. *Lazarus Is Dead*. New York: Europa Editions, 2012.

Blanke, Charles Michael LeBlanc, Dawn Hershman, Lee Ellis, and Frank Meyskens. "Characterizing 18 Years of the Death with Dignity Act in Oregon." *JAMA Oncology* 3 (2017): 1403–6. https://doi.org/10.1001/jamaoncol.2017.0243.

Braverman, Derek W., Brian S. Marcus, Paul G. Wakim, Mark R. Mercurio, and Gary S. Kopf. "Health Care Professionals' Attitudes about Physician-Assisted Death: An Analysis of Their Justifications and the Roles of Terminology and Patient Competency." *Journal of Pain and Symptom Management* 54 (2017): 538–45. https://doi.org/10.1016/j.jpainsymman.2017.07.024.

Byock, Ira. *Dying Well: The Prospect for Growth at the End of Life*. New York: Riverhead Books, 1997.

Cantor, Norman L. *After We Die: The Life and Times of the Human Cadaver*. Washington, DC: Georgetown University Press, 2010.

Carr, Deborah. "'I Don't Want to Die Like That . . .': The Impact of Significant Others' Death Quality on Advance Care Planning." *Gerontologist* 52 (2012): 770–81.

Cassell, Eric J. *The Nature of Suffering and the Goals of Medicine*. Oxford: Oxford University Press, 1991.

Cheung, Gary, Gwendolyn Douwes, and Frederick Sundram. "Late-Life Suicide in Terminal Cancer: A Rational Act or Underdiagnosed Depression?" *Journal of Pain and Symptom Management* 54 (2017): 835–42. https://doi.org/10.1016/j.jpainsymman.2017.05.004.

Chochinov, Harvey Max, Linda J. Kristjanson, William Breitbart, Susan McClement, Thomas F. Hack, Tom Hassard, and Mike Harlos. "The Effect of Dignity Therapy on Distress and End-of-Life Experience in Terminally Ill Patients: A Randomised Controlled Trial." *Lancet Oncology* 12 (2011): 753–62.

The Conversation Project. "Starter Kits." Accessed November 20, 2019. https://www.theconversationproject.org/starter-kits.

Daudet, Alphonse. *In the Land of Pain.* Edited and translated by Julian Barnes. New York: Alfred A. Knopf, 2002.

Death Cafe. Accessed November 20, 2019. https://deathcafe.com.

DeMartino, Erin S., David M. Dudzinski, Cavan K. Doyle, Beau P. Sperry, Sarah E. Gregor, Mark Siegler, Daniel P. Sulmasy, Paul S. Mueller, and Daniel B. Kramer. "Who Decides When a Patient Can't? Statutes on Alternate Decision Makers." *New England Journal of Medicine* 376 (2017): 1478–82. https://doi.org/10.1056/NEJMms1611497.

Department of Health and Human Services. "Hospice Compare." Accessed November 10, 2019. https://www.medicare.gov/hospicecompare.

Department of Health and Human Services. "Medicare and Medicaid Programs: Hospice Conditions of Participation." June 5, 2008. Accessed June 13, 2018. https://www.govinfo.gov/content/pkg/FR-2008-06-05/pdf/08-1305.pdf.

Dorje, Gyurme, trans. *The Tibetan Book of the Dead.* Edited by Graham Coleman with Thupten Jinpa. New York: Viking, 2005.

Dostoevsky, Fyodor. *The Idiot.* Translated by Anna Brailovsky. New York: Modern Library, 2003.

Emanuel, Linda L., Neha Reddy, Joshua Hauser, and Sarah B. Sonnenfeld. "'And Yet It Was a Blessing': The Case for Existential Maturity." *Journal of Palliative Medicine* 20 (2017): 318–27.

Evans-Wentz, W. Y., trans. and ed. *The Tibetan Book of the Dead.* London: Oxford University Press, 1927.

Finucane, Thomas E., Colleen Christmas, and Kathy Travis. "Tube Feeding in Patients with Advanced Dementia: A Review of the Evidence." *Journal of the American Medical Association* 282 (1999): 1365–70. https://doi.org/10.1001/jama.282.14.1365.

Ganzini, Linda, Elizabeth R. Goy, Lois L. Miller, Theresa A. Harvath, Ann Jackson, and Molly A. Delorit. "Nurses' Experiences with Hospice Patients Who Refuse Food and Fluids to Hasten Death." *New England Journal of Medicine* 349 (2003): 359–65. https://doi.org/10.1056/NEJMsa035086.

Garrido, Melissa M., Ellen L. Idler, Howard Leventhal, and Deborah Carr. "Pathways from Religion to Advance Care Planning: Beliefs about Control over Length of Life and End-of-Life Values." *Gerontologist* 53 (2013): 801–16. https://doi.org/10.1093/geront/gns128.

Gawande, Atul. *Being Mortal: Medicine and What Matters in the End.* New York: Metropolitan Books, 2014.

Gostin, Lawrence O. "Ethics, the Constitution, and the Dying Process: The Case of Theresa Marie Schiavo." *Journal of the American Medical Association* 293 (2005): 2403–7. https://doi.org/10.1001/jama.293.19.2403.

Hawley, Jack. *The Bhagavad Gita: A Walkthrough for Westerners.* Novato, CA: New World Library, 2001.

Hemingway, Ernest. *For Whom the Bell Tolls.* New York: Simon & Schuster, 1940.

Jacobs, Lenworth M., Karyl Burns, and Barbara Bennett Jacobs. "Trauma Death: Views of the Public and Trauma Professionals on Death and Dying from Injuries." *Archives of Surgery* 143 (2008): 730–35. https://doi.org/10.1001/archsurg.143.8.730.

Johnson, Philip G. "Raleigh Seminarian with Terminal Brain Cancer Responds to Brittany Maynard." Catholic Diocese of Raleigh. Accessed November 10, 2019. https://dioceseofraleigh.org/news/raleigh-seminarian-terminal-brain-cancer-responds-brittany-maynard.

Karner, Maggie. "Brain Cancer Will Likely Kill Me, but There's No Way I'll Kill Myself." TheFederalist.com, October 10, 2014. Accessed November 10, 2019. https://thefederalist.com/2014/10/10/brain-cancer-will-likely-kill-me-but-theres-no-way-ill-kill-myself.

Kempis, Thomas à. *The Imitation of Christ*. New York: Grosset and Dunlap, 1973.

Kochanek, Kenneth D., Sherry L. Murphy, Jiaquan Xu, and Elizabeth Arias. "Deaths: Final Data for 2017." *National Vital Statistics Reports* 68 (2019). https://www.cdc.gov/nchs/data/nvsr/nvsr68/nvsr68_09-508.pdf.

Koopman, J. J. E., and H. Putter. "Regional Variation in the Practice of Euthanasia and Physician-Assisted Suicide in the Netherlands." *Netherlands Journal of Medicine* 74 (2016): 387–94. http://www.njmonline.nl/article.php?a=1777&d=1181&i=200.

Kouwenhoven, Pauline S. C., Natasja J. H. Raijmakers, Johannes J. M. van Delden, Judith A. C. Rietjens, Donald G. van Tol, Suzanne van de Vathorst, Neinke de Graeff, Heleen A. M. Weyers, Agnes van der Heide, and Ghislaine J. M. W. van Thiel. "Opinions about Euthanasia and Advanced Dementia: A Qualitative Study among Dutch Physicians and Members of the General Public." *BMC Medical Ethics* 16, no. 7 (2015). https://doi.org/10.1186/1472-6939-16-7.

Maynard, Brittany. "My Right to Death with Dignity at 29." Accessed November 10, 2019. https://compassionandchoices.org/stories/brittany-maynard.

McCue, Jack D. "Freud's Physician-Assisted Death." *Archives of Internal Medicine* 159 (1999): 1521–25. https://doi.org/10.1001/archinte.159.14.1521.

McNally, Bryan, Rachel Robb, Monica Mehta, Kimberly Vellano, Amy L. Valderrama, Paula W. Yoon, Comilla Sassoon, Allison Crouch, Amanda Bray Perez, Robert Merritt, and Arthur Kellerman. "Out-of-Hospital Cardiac Arrest Surveillance—Cardiac Arrest Registry to Enhance Survival (CARES), United States, October 1, 2005–December 31, 2010." *Morbidity and Mortality Weekly Report Surveillance Summaries* 60 (2011): 1–19. https://www.cdc.gov/mmwr/preview/mmwrhtml/ss6008a1.htm?s_cid=ss6008a1_w.

Mercadente, Sebastiano, Giuseppe Intravaia, Patrizia Villari, Patrizia Ferrera, Fabrizio David, and Alessandra Casuccio. "Controlled Sedation for Refractory Symptoms in Dying Patients." *Journal of Pain and Symptom Management* 37 (2009): 771–79. https://doi.org/10.1016/j.jpainsymman.2008.04.020.

Milton, John. *Paradise Lost*. New York: Oxford University Press, 2005.

Oregon Health Authority. "Oregon Death with Dignity Act: 2018 Data Summary." Accessed November 10, 2019. https://www.oregon.gov/oha/PH/PROVIDERPARTNERRESOURCES/EVALUATIONRESEARCH/DEATHWITHDIGNITYACT/Documents/year21.pdf.

Oregon Health Authority. "Oregon Revised Statute: Oregon's Death with Dignity Act." Accessed November 10, 2019. https://www.oregon.gov/oha/PH/PROVIDERPARTNERRESOURCES/EVALUATIONRESEARCH/DEATHWITHDIGNITYACT/Pages/ors.aspx.

Ostaseski, Frank. *The Five Invitations: Discovering What Death Can Teach Us about Living Fully*. New York: Flat Iron Books, 2017.

Penn, William. *Some Fruits of Solitude*. Accessed November 18, 2019. https://www.bartleby.com/1/3/170.html.

Phelps, Andrea C., Paul K. Maciejewski, Matthew Nilsson, Tracy A. Balboni, Alexi A. Wright, M. Elizabeth Paulk, Elizabeth Trice, Deborah Schrag, John R. Peteet, Susan D. Block, and Holly G. Prigerson. "Religious Coping and Use of Intensive

Life-Prolonging Care Near Death in Patients with Advanced Cancer." *Journal of the American Medical Association* 301 (2009): 1140–47. https://doi.org/10.1001/jama.2009.341.

Plato. *The Last Days of Socrates*. Translated by Hugh Tredennick and Harold Tarant. London: Penguin Books, 2003.

Plato. *The Republic*. Translated by Benjamin Jowett. New York: Modern Library, 1941.

Presbyterian Church (USA), 345. "A Brief Statement of Faith." Accessed November 10, 2019. http://oga.pcusa.org/site_media/media/uploads/oga/pdf/boc2016.pdf.

Riley, James Whitcomb. "Little Orphant Annie." In *The Family Album of Favorite Poems*, edited by P. Edward Ernest, 493–94. New York: Grosset and Dunlap, 1959.

Roach, Mary. *Stiff: The Curious Lives of Human Cadavers*. New York: W. W. Norton, 2003.

Ruijs, Cees D. M., Gerrit van der Wal, Ad J. F. M. Kerkhof, and Bregje D. Onwutea-ka-Philipsen. "Unbearable Suffering and Requests for Euthanasia Prospectively Studied in End-of-Life Cancer Patients in Primary Care." *BMC Palliative Care* 13 (2014). https://doi.org/10.1186/1472-684X-13-62.

Sandomir, Richard. "Raymond Smullyan, Puzzle-Creating Logician, Dies at 97." *New York Times*, February 11, 2017. https://www.nytimes.com/2017/02/11/us/raymond-smullyan-dead-puzzle-creator.html.

Saunders, Cecily E. Foreword to *Oxford Textbook of Palliative Medicine*, 3rd ed., edited by Derek Doyle, Geoffrey Hanks, Nathan Cherny, and Kenneth Calman, xvii–xx. Oxford: Oxford University Press, 2004.

Selmanovic, Samir. "If Muhammad Had Not Spoken." In *My Neighbor's Faith: Stories of Interreligious Encounter, Growth, and Transformation*, edited by Jennifer Howe Peace, Or N. Rose, and Gregory Mobley, 211–13. Maryknoll, NY: Orbis Books, 2012.

Shankaran, Veena, Richard J. LaFrance, and Scott D. Ramsey. "Drug Price Inflation and the Cost of Assisted Death for Terminally Ill Patients—Death with Indignity." *JAMA Oncology* 3 (2017): 15–16. https://doi.org/10.1001/jamaoncol.2016.3842.

Steinhauser, Karen E., Nicholas A. Christakis, Elizabeth C. Clipp, Maya McNeilly, Lauren McIntyre, and James A. Tulsky. "Factors Considered Important at the End of Life by Patients, Family, Physicians, and Other Care Providers." *Journal of the American Medical Association* 284 (2000): 2476–82. https://doi.org/10.1001/jama.284.19.2476.

The SUPPORT Principal Investigators. "A Controlled Trial to Improve Care for Seriously Ill Hospitalized Patients: The Study to Understand Prognoses and Preferences for Outcomes and Risks of Treatments (SUPPORT)." *Journal of the American Medical Association* 274 (1995): 1591–98. https://doi.org/10.1001/jama.1995.03530200027032.

Temel, Jennifer S., Joseph A. Greer, Alona Muzikansky, Emily R. Gallagher, Sonal Admane, Vicki A. Jackson, Constance M. Dahlin, Craig D. Blinderman, Juliet Jacobsen, William F. Pirl, J. Andrew Billings, and Thomas J. Lynch. "Early Palliative Care for Patients with Metastatic Non-Small-Cell Lung Cancer." *New England Journal of Medicine* 363 (2010): 733–42. https://doi.org/10.1056/NEJMoa1000678.

Teno, Joan M., Pedro Gozalo, Amal N. Trivedi, Jennifer Bunker, Julie Lima, Jessica Ogarek, and Vincent Mor. "Site of Death, Place of Care, and Health Care Transitions among US Medicare Beneficiaries, 2000–2015." *Journal of the American Medical Association* 320 (2018): 264–71. https://doi.org/10.1001/jama.2018.8981.

Theroux, Paul. "D Is for Death." In *Hockney's Alphabet*, by David Hockney, edited by Stephen Spender. New York: Random House, 1991.

Tippett, Krista. *Becoming Wise: An Inquiry into the Mystery and Art of Living*. New York: Penguin Books, 2016.

Toll, Susan, and Joan M. Teno. "Lessons from Oregon in Embracing Complexity in End-of-Life Care." *New England Journal of Medicine* 376 (2017): 1078–82. https://doi.org/10.1056/NEJMsb1612511.

Tolstoy, Leo. "The Death of Ivan Ilych." In *The Death of Ivan Ilych and Other Stories*, translated by Rosemary Edmonds, 99–161. London: Penguin Books, 1960.

Twain, Mark. *The Adventures of Tom Sawyer*. New York: Penguin, 2014.

Twain, Mark. *The Autobiography of Mark Twain*. New York: Harper & Row, 2010.

Zitter, Jessica Nutik. *Extreme Measures: Finding a Better Path to the End of Life*. New York: Avery, 2017.

INDEX

ABOUT THE AUTHOR

Dr. Jeff Spiess is "mostly" retired as associate medical director of Hospice of the Western Reserve. He has spent his medical career caring for those facing serious illness and death, first as an oncologist then as a hospice physician, and he has been recognized as a leader in his field. His previous publications have included scholarly articles and reflective narratives. His interest in theology and spirituality inform both his writing and his approach to the care of his patients.